Costume at Castle Howard

Printed in England ISBN 0 9502545 2 5

Introduction

This picture book is not intended to be yet one more history of costume, of which there are many excellent examples. Its purpose is to illustrate in chronological order some of the more attractive or interesting dresses and other costumes from the collection at Castle Howard. All but two of the photographs were taken against the backdrop of Castle Howard and its surroundings.
The period costumes housed and shown in the Stables at Castle Howard form the largest private collection in Britain. Only a very small proportion is shown at any one time: the display, in realistic settings, is changed each winter, which allows us not only to put on exhibition a different selection annually, but also to pay the maximum attention to the conservation of those costumes which are not on show. Above all, it means that no fabric is exposed to light for long periods, light being, generally, the most dangerous threat to the majority of textiles.
The Costume Galleries were founded in 1965. The Stables had been empty of horses, except for an occasional pony, for 50 years: during the 1950s they had housed cows and, later, potatoes, but I was anxious to find a more suitable use than this for the fine range of buildings, which had been designed by John Carr in 1782. At the same time Miss Cecile Hummel was looking for a home for the collection of costumes which she had formed, examples of which she was using as illustrations for her lectures. We met: her collection moved to Castle Howard, with her as curator, and we opened our first display to the public in 1965 as an additional attraction to the house itself, which has been open ever since it was built in the early 1700s. Within a few years gifts and loans to the Castle Howard collection greatly outnumbered the original items, and some gaps were filled by a small number of purchases. Outstanding amongst these were ballet

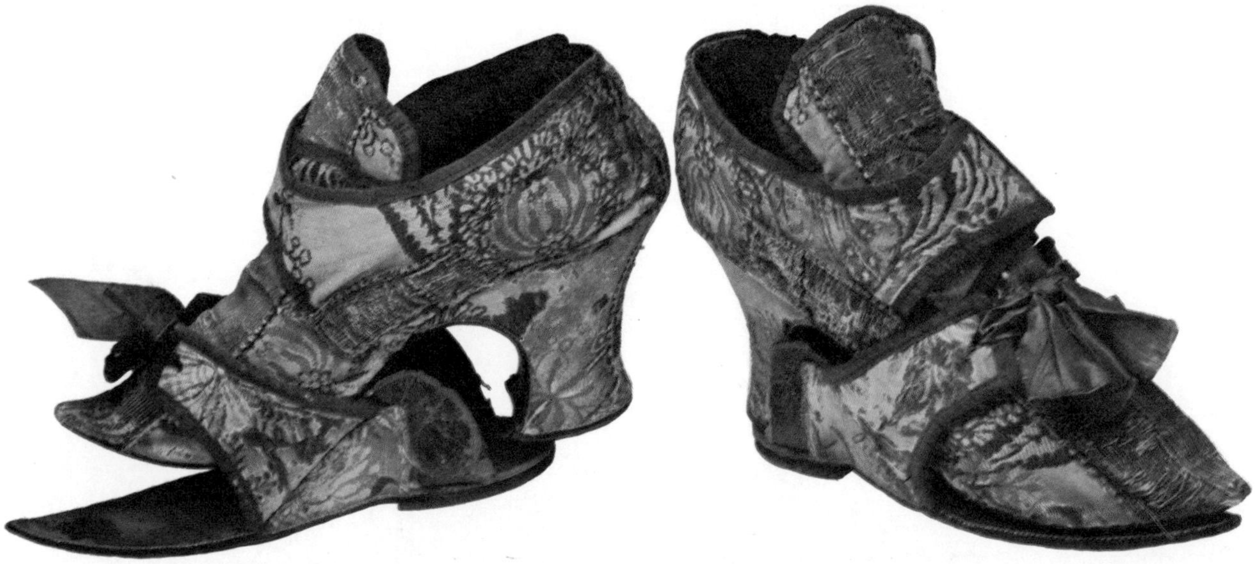

costumes acquired at the dispersals of the Diaghilev Ballet Company wardrobe. We possess costumes for 10 ballets, including those designed by Matisse for Le Chant du Rossignol, by Bakst for The Sleeping Princess and by Roerich for Le Sacre du Printemps.

The earliest item in the collection is the buff coat worn by General Fairfax, the Cromwellian commander, which still retains its original silver braid and pink lining. Other 17th and early 18th century items are sparse, but from then on most periods are represented, right through to the present day; the collection is kept up-to-date by the accession of examples of the latest fashions.

Miss Hummel retired after 9 arduous and fruitful years, during which the Costume Galleries were firmly set on their present course; our warmest thanks are due to her for her unstinting and imaginative labours in the display and understanding of the whole field of Costume. She was succeeded as Curator by Richard Robson.

I am grateful to the Department of Textiles at the Victoria and Albert Museum, for their assistance in checking the accuracy of dates and other facts, though I must, of course, bear full responsibility for any mistakes. My special thanks are due to Beatrice Dawson for help given so generously from her unrivalled experience in costume design.

The Galleries are meant to be enjoyed, as well as being used by students of costume and social history: I hope that the same can be said of this book.

This book is dedicated to the memory of C., my partner in all things for 25 years; she loved beautiful clothes, and without her the Costume Galleries would not have existed.

George Howard

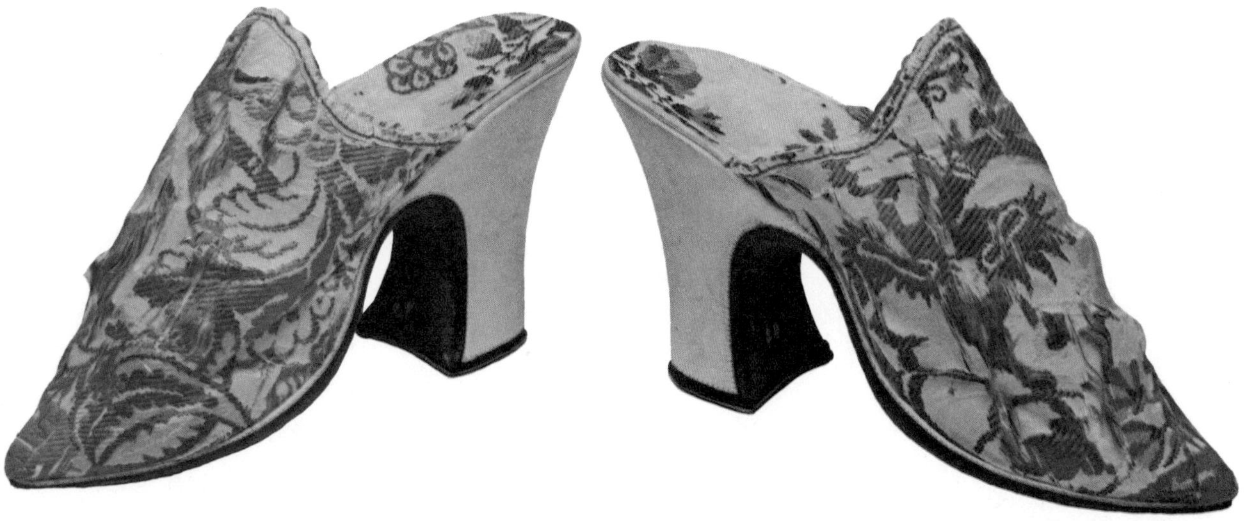

The first 50 years of the 18th century had seen men vieing with women in the flamboyance of their costume, but by 1770 men's clothing at least began to adopt more restrained lines and colour, as can be seen in this French waistcoat of about 1785 with its floral designs and buttons on a neutral background. The group on the facing page is of the same period, and shows, from left to right, a woven French silk dress, a man's silver embroidered cut velvet jacket with an embroidered waistcoat, a boy's pink and cream suit, and a sacque dress of heavy woven silk, trimmed with lace and flowers. This can be seen in more detail on the next page, illustrating clearly the intricacies of pattern common to ladies' dresses of this time.

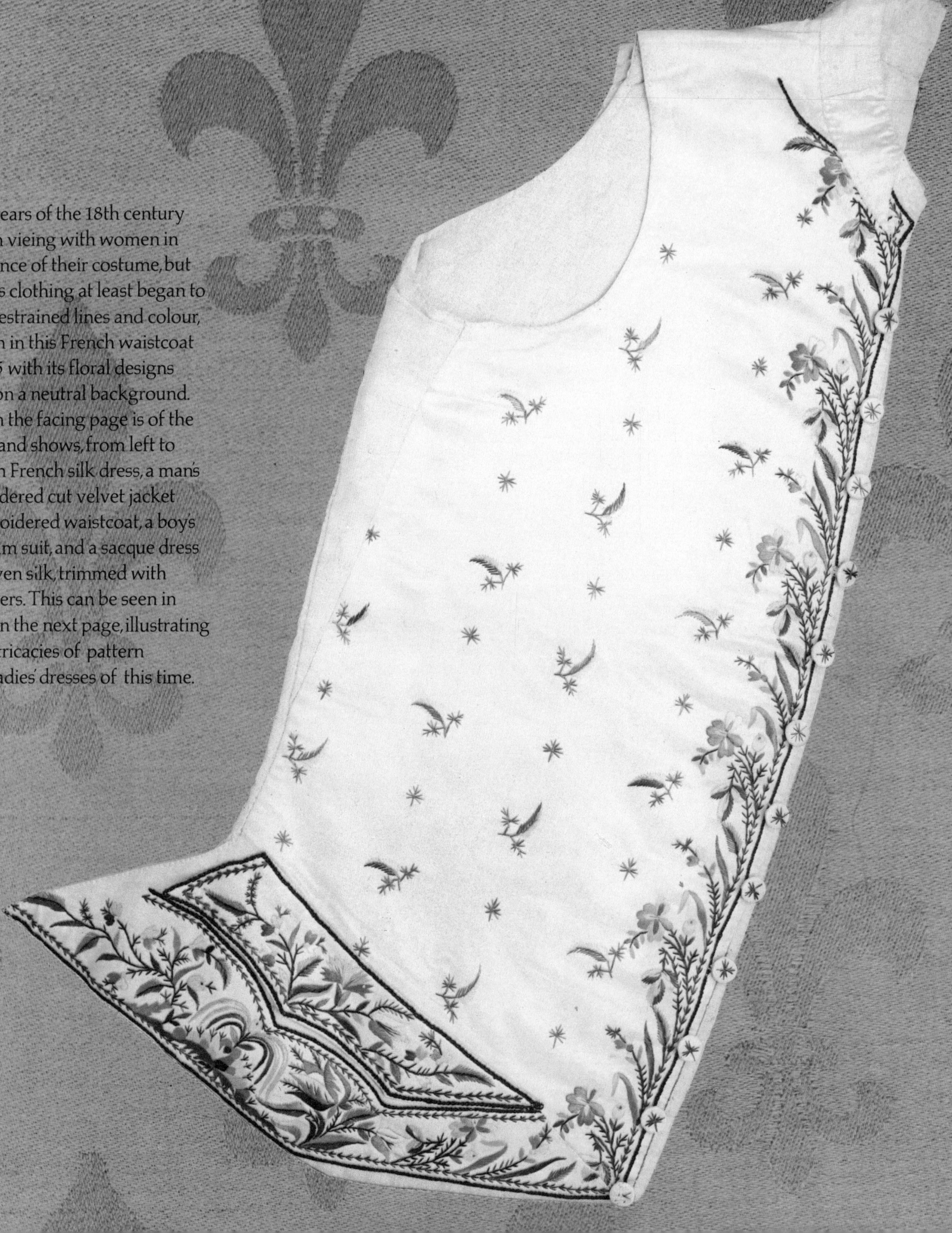

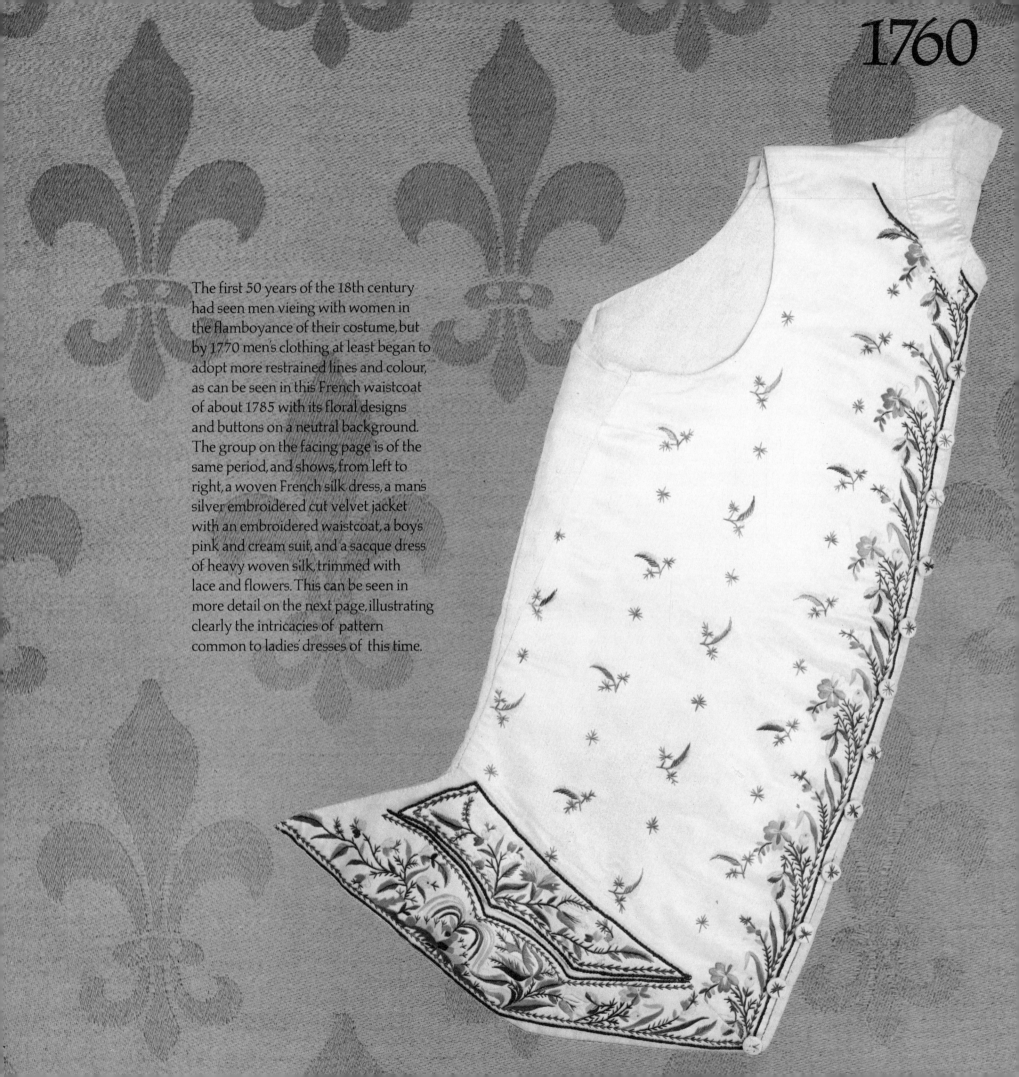

1785

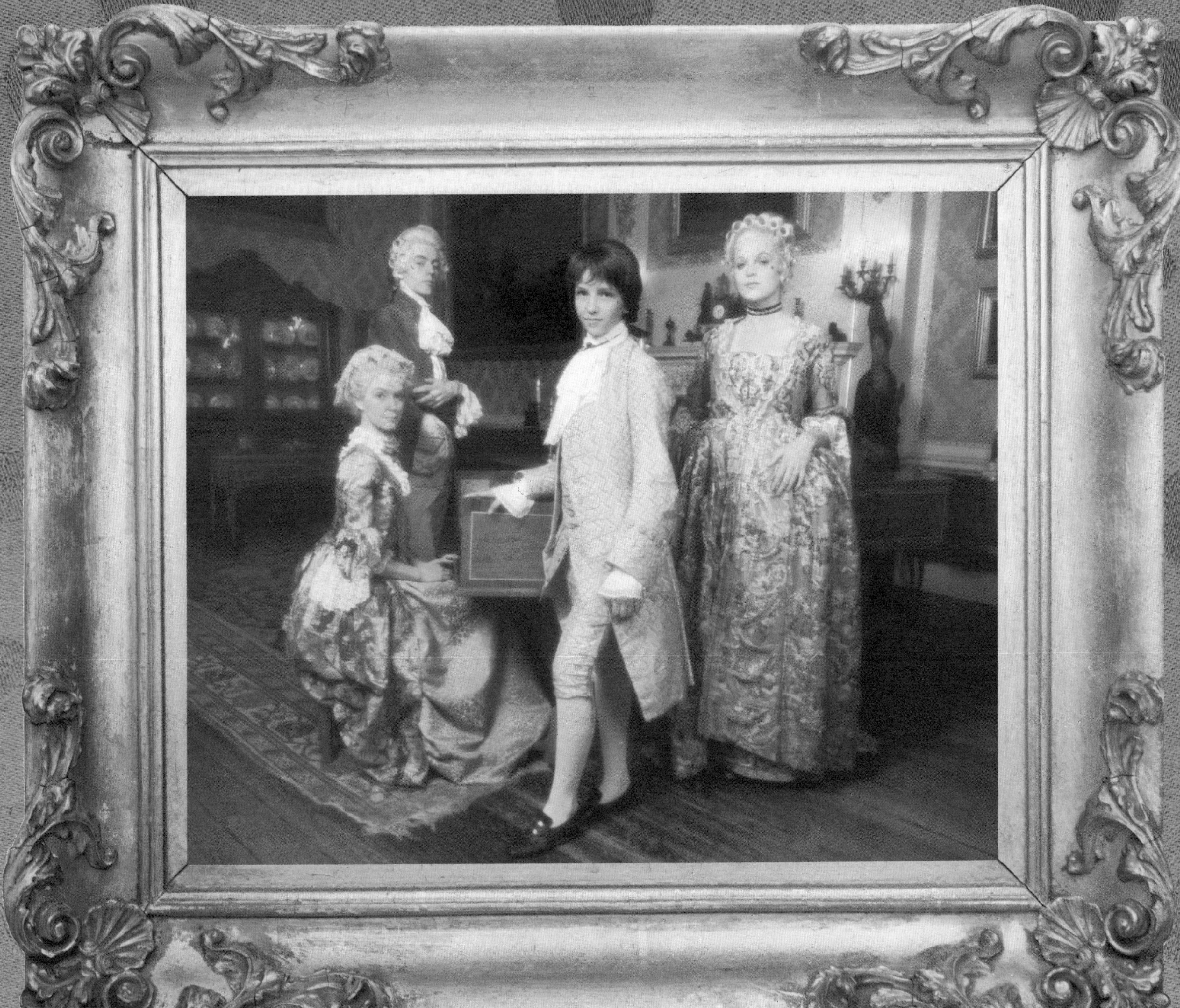

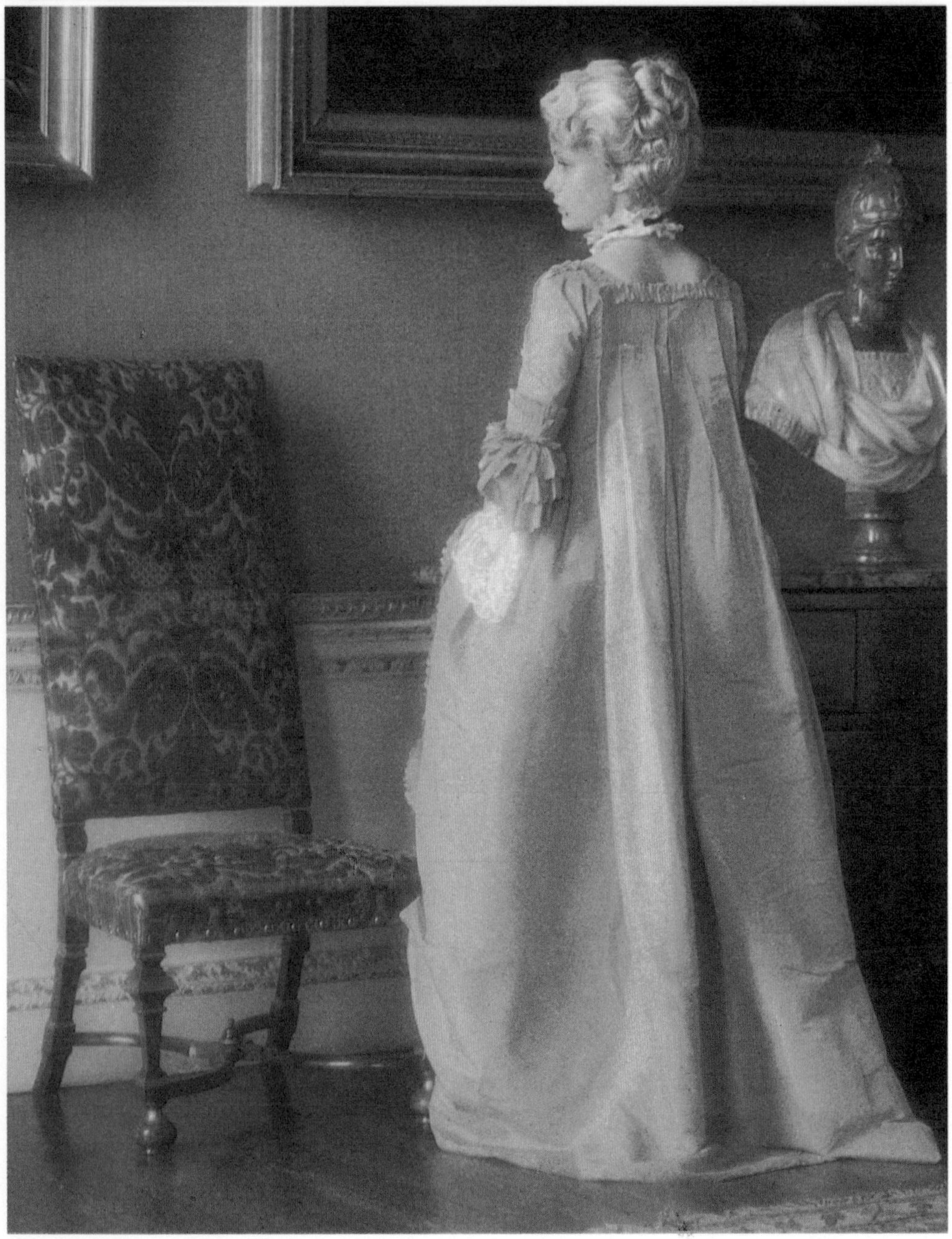

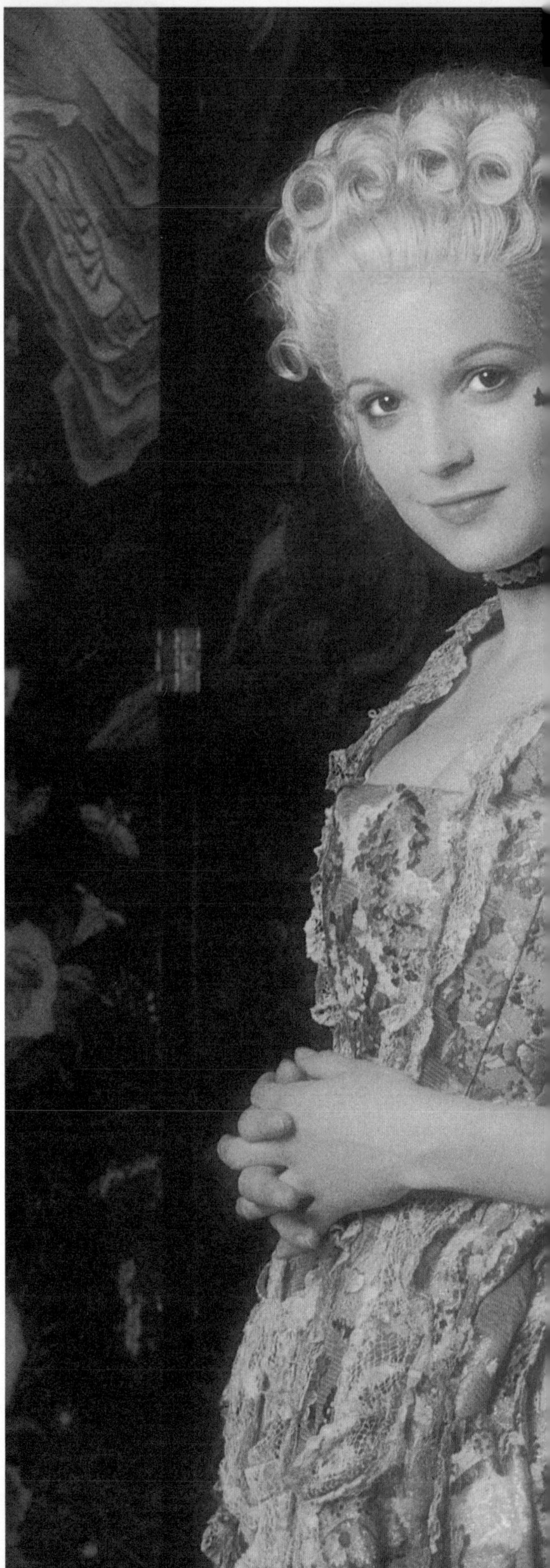

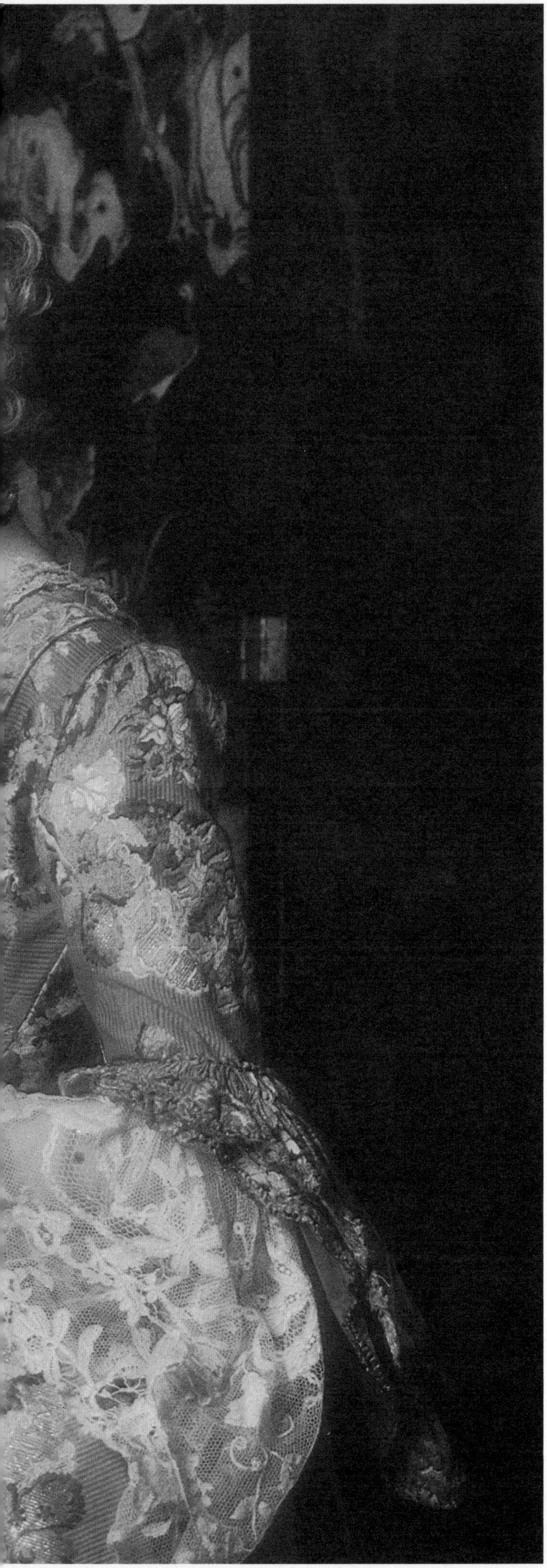

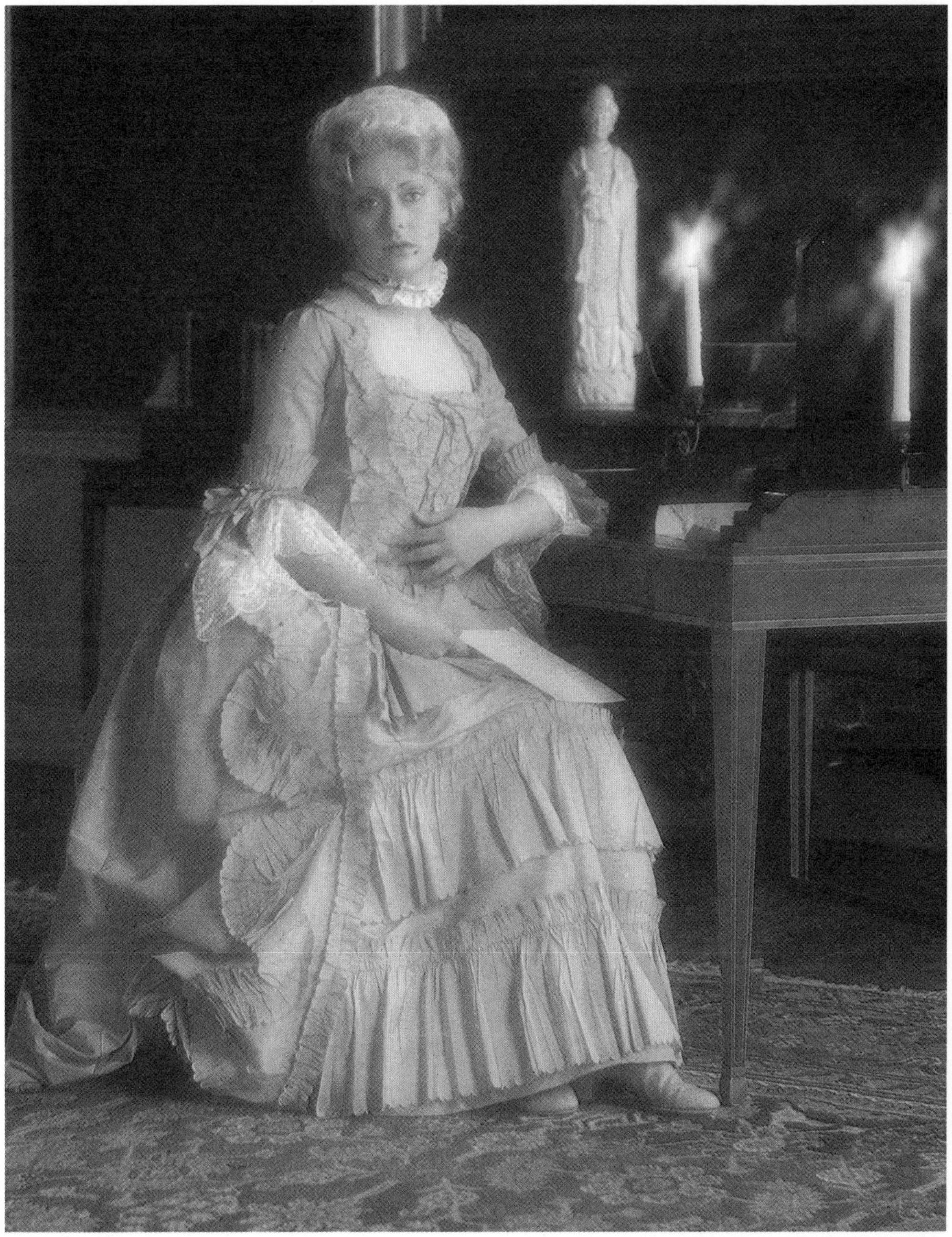

1765 A predominant form of 18th century dress was the sacque backed gown, with flowing back and fitting front; the examples shown are in yellow taffeta, trimmed with scalloped self silk, and in heavy woven silk trimmed with lace and flowers.

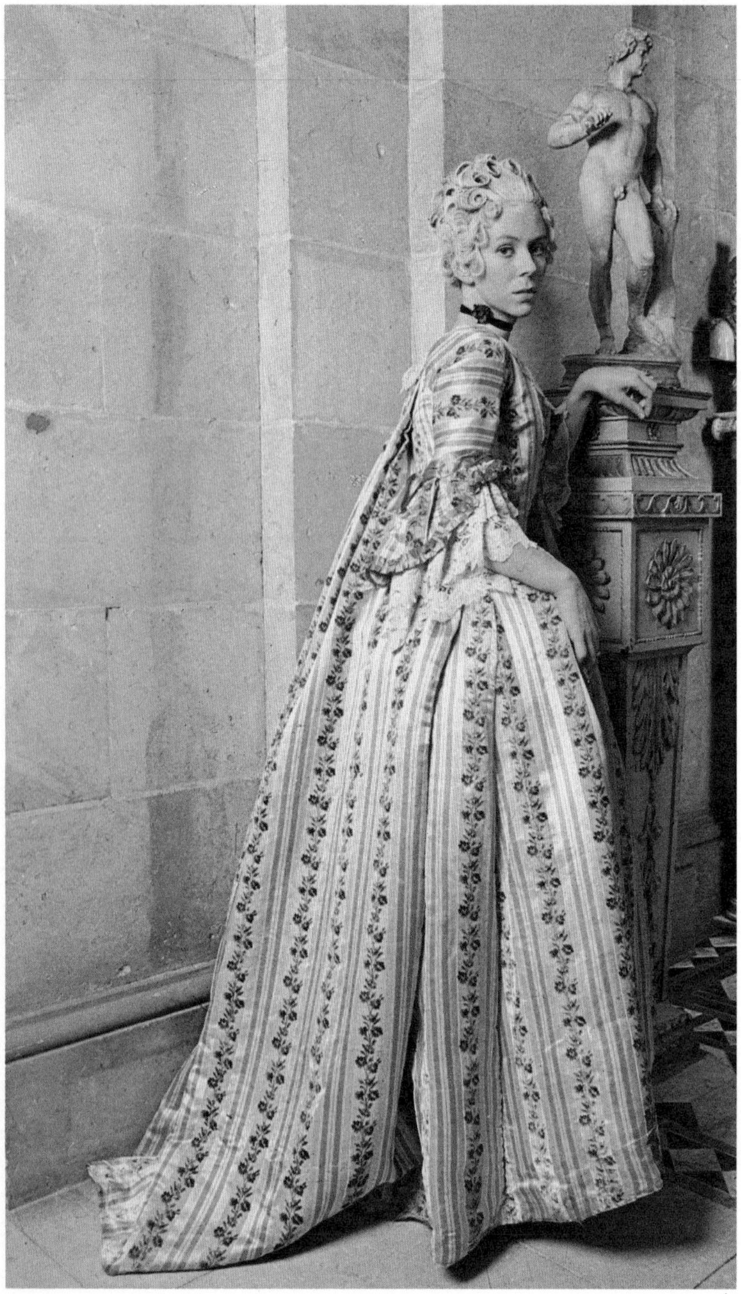

1774

This is a particularly fascinating sacque back dress of 1774; the material, called chiné, was woven as one piece, in striped satin and flowered velvet, but sadly, the process was lost at the time of the French Revolution.

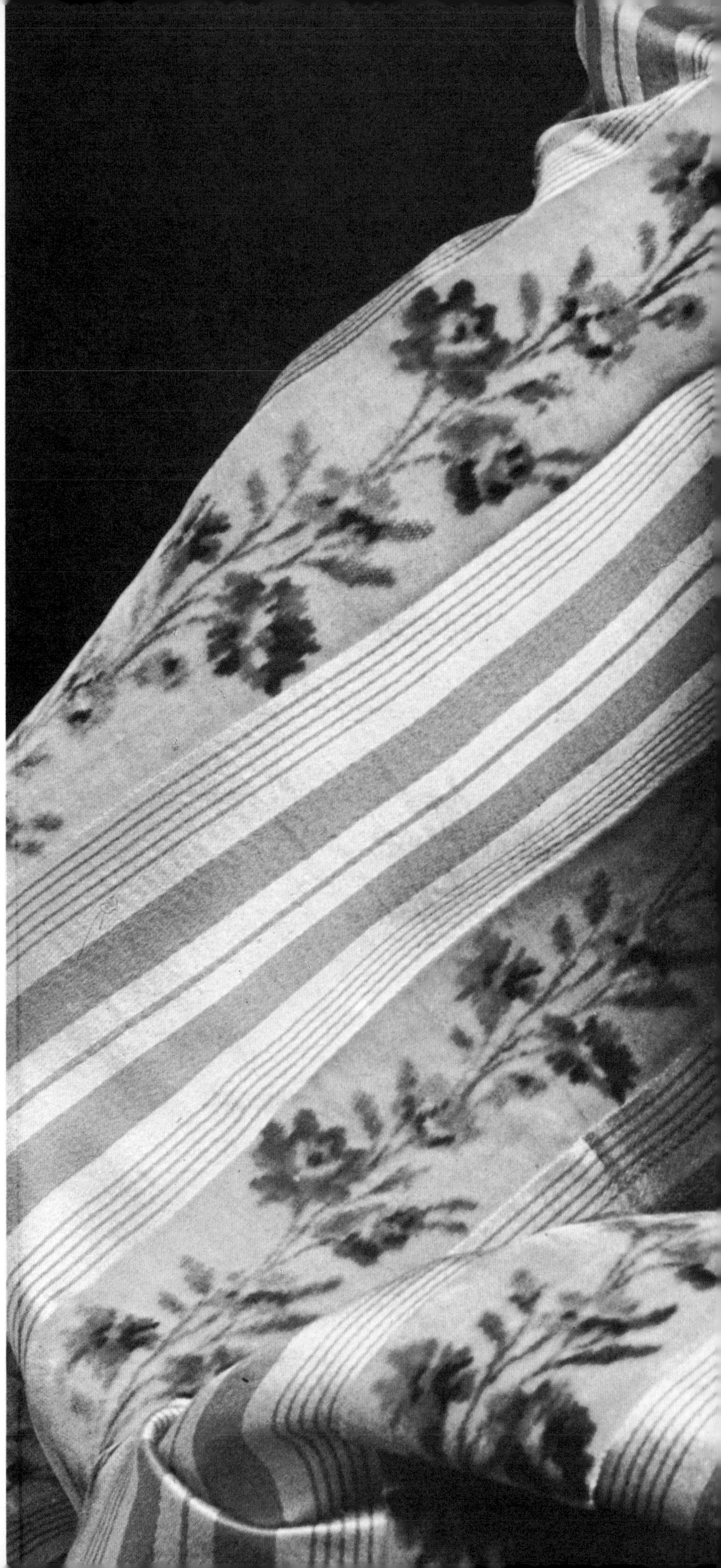

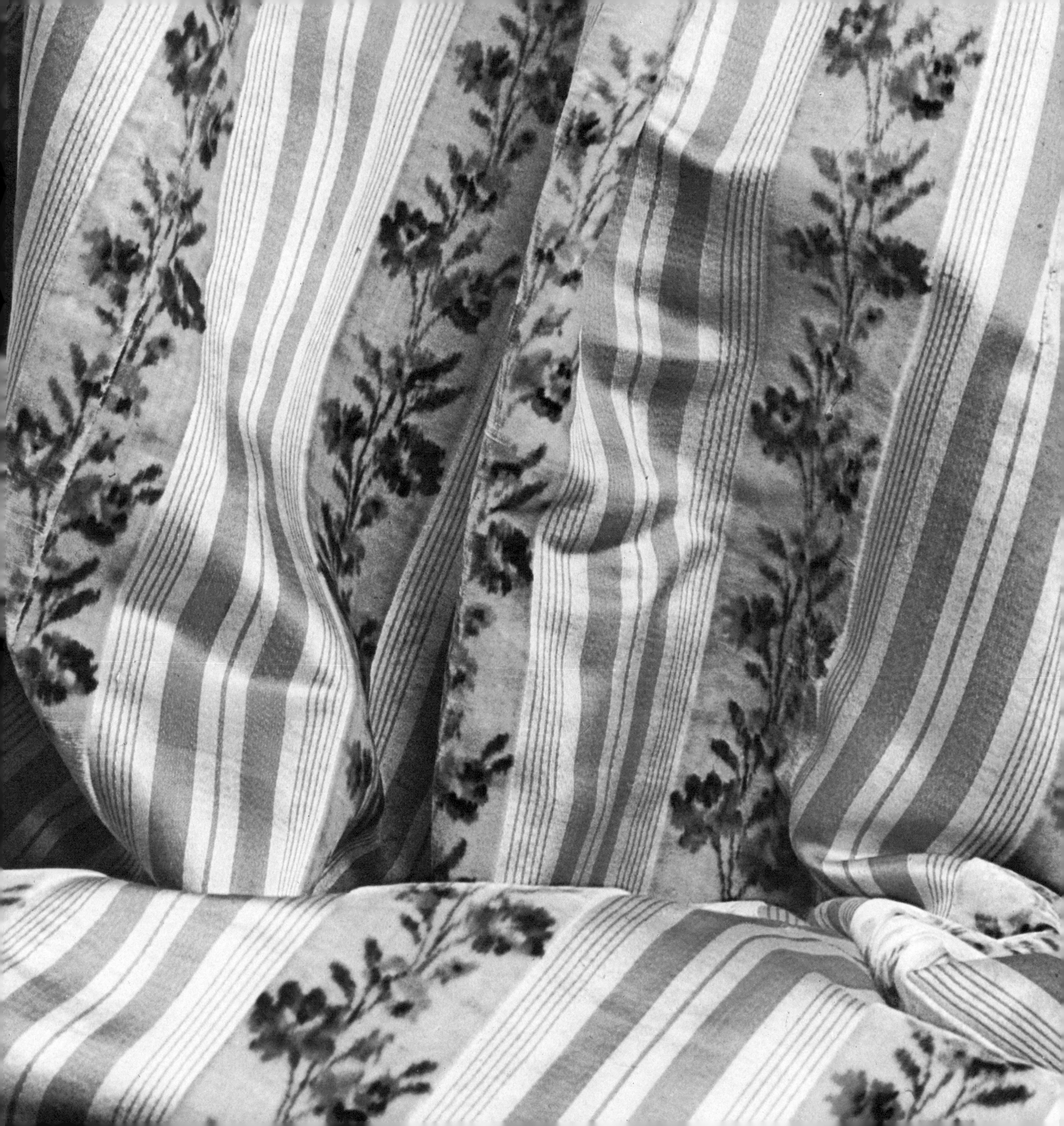

1806

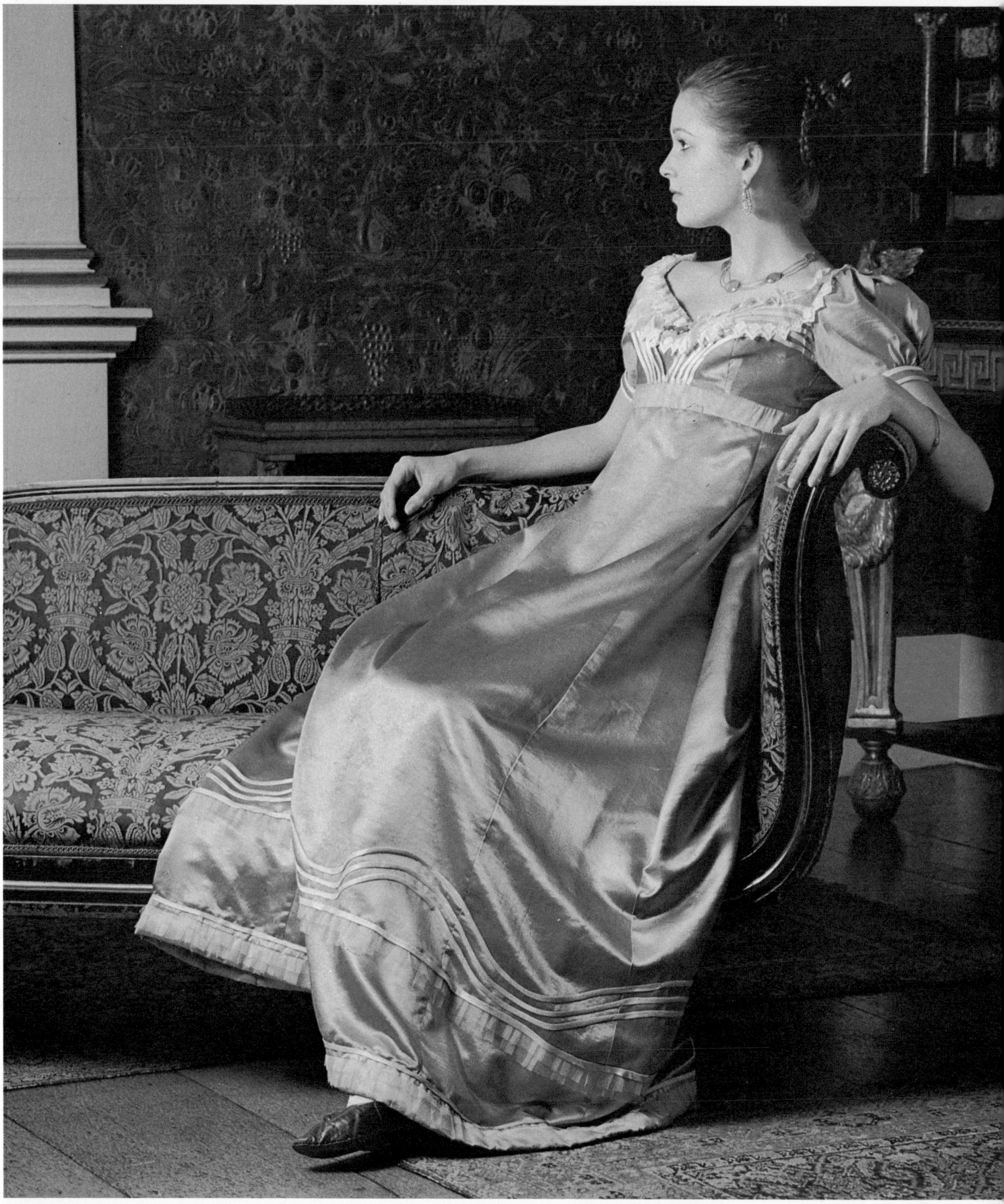

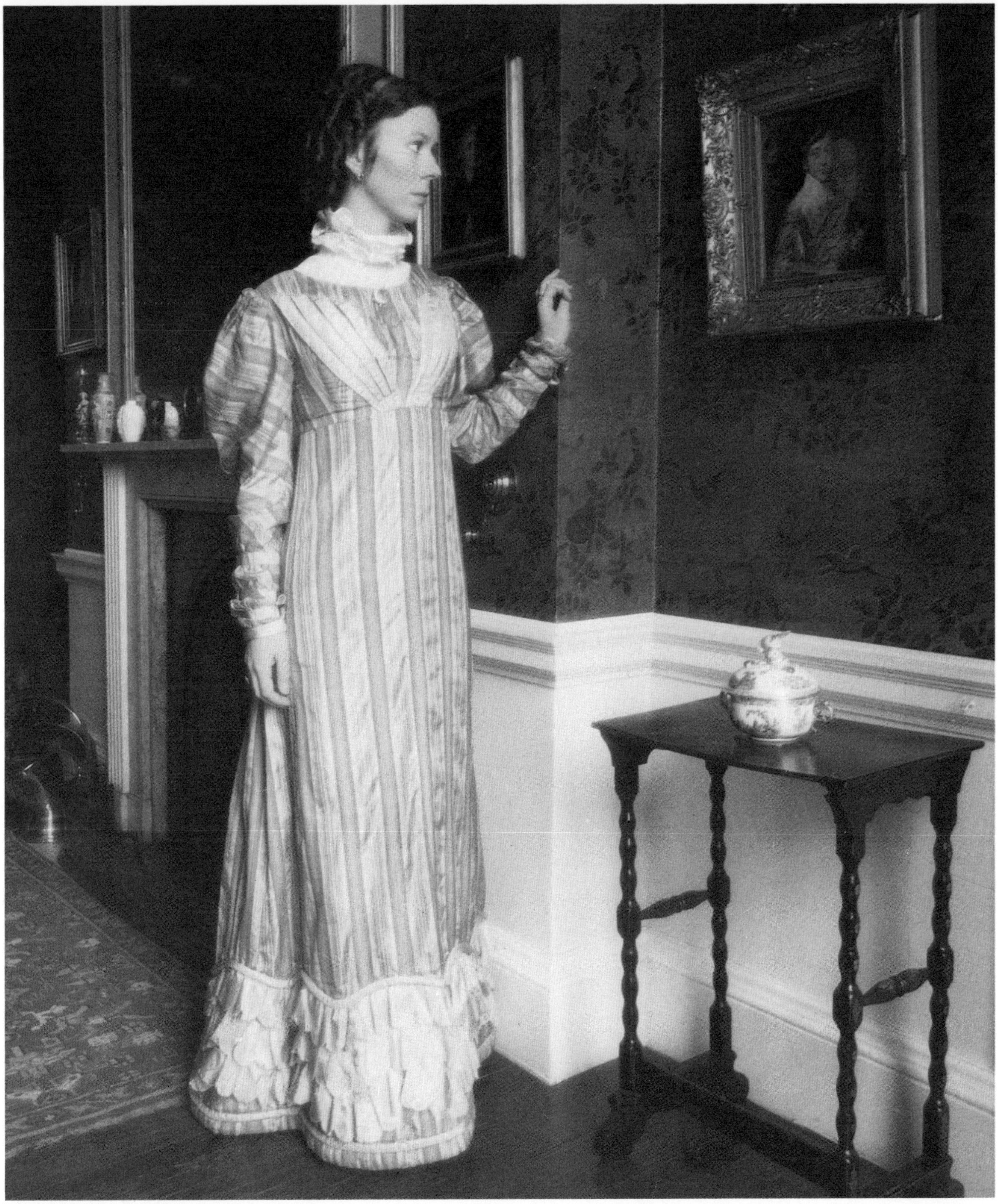

1827

As this yellow-gold satin evening dress of 1806 shows, the Revolution brought about great changes in fashion; gone are the billowing petticoats, panniers and vice-like corsets of the 18th century, to be replaced by the simpler, pseudo-classical lines of the French Empire.

The whole dress is now one piece, in contrast to the skirts and tops of previous years. But by the time the blue striped day dress was made, in 1827, elaboration of design was returning; the pinked frills at the hem, wider, longer sleeves and a high neck line all point to a swing away from the simplicity of the previous twenty years.

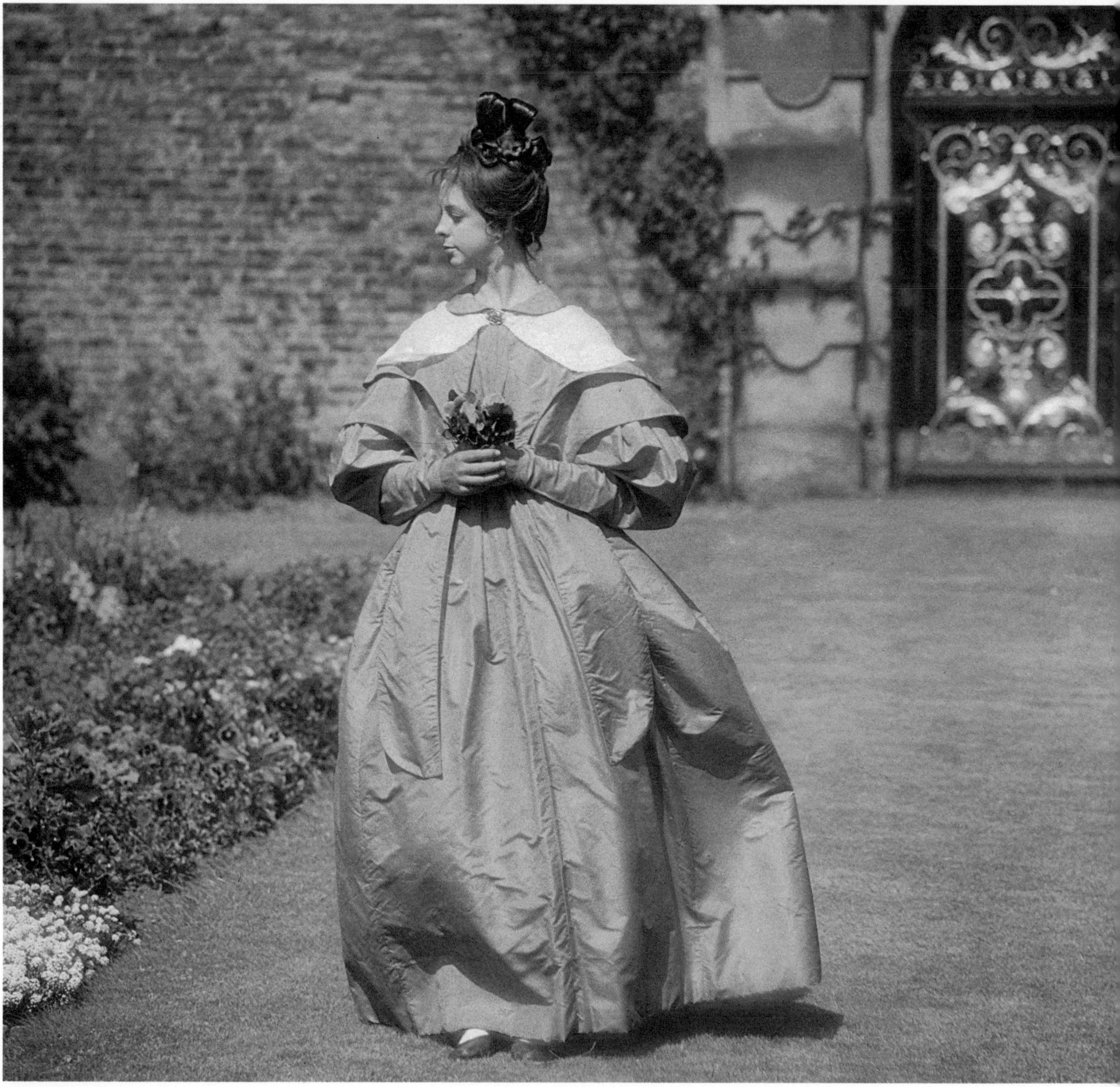

1835 Salient features of this period are the leg of mutton (gigot) sleeves, the widening skirt, and the addition of a small top garment, such as the pellerine on this beige silk dress of 1835.

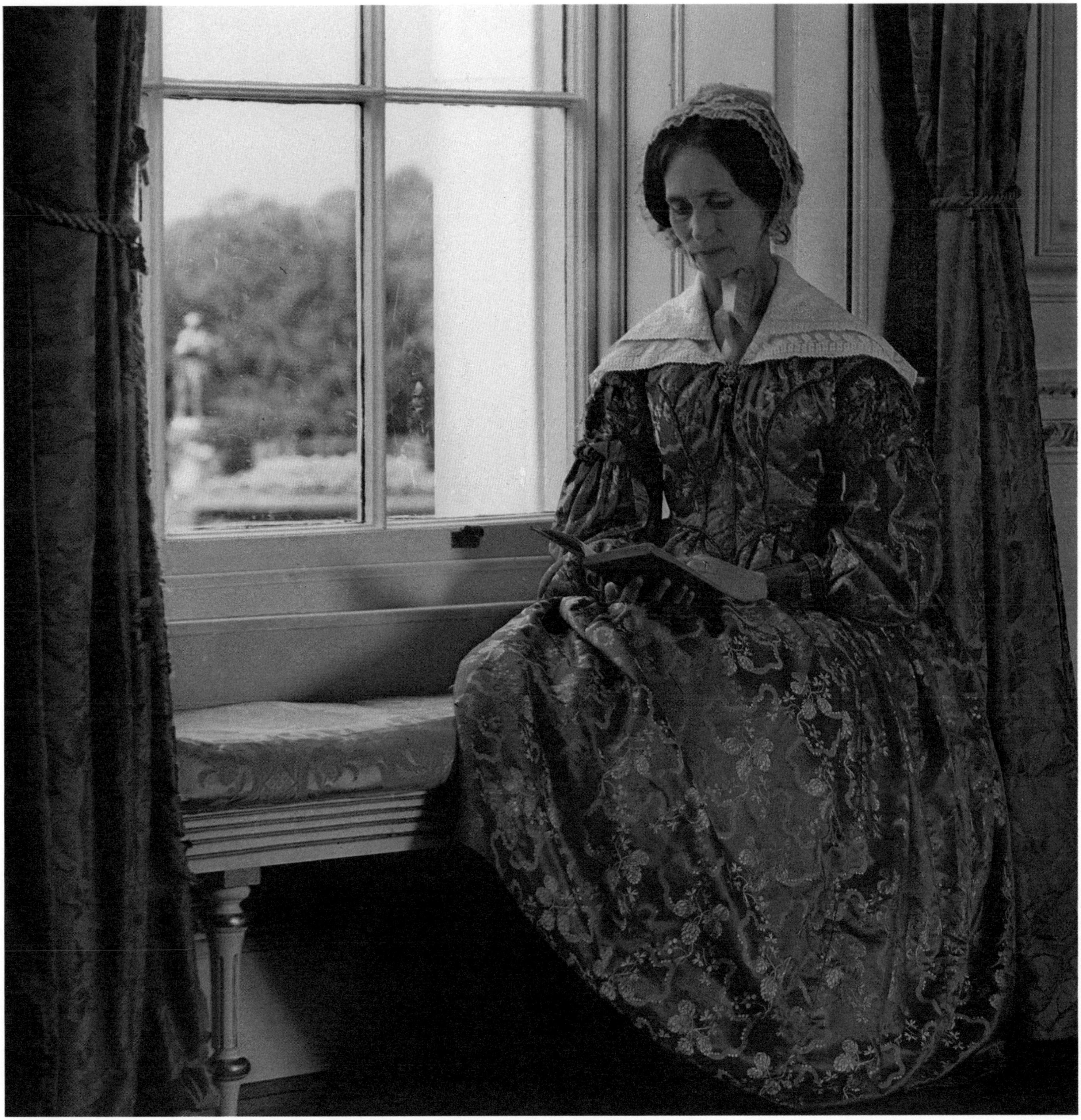

1836

While more complex patterns begin to appear in the materials used, as in this silk brocade dress of the same date, the trimmings remain simple, being no more than a lawn neck covering and a muslin cap in this case.

1838

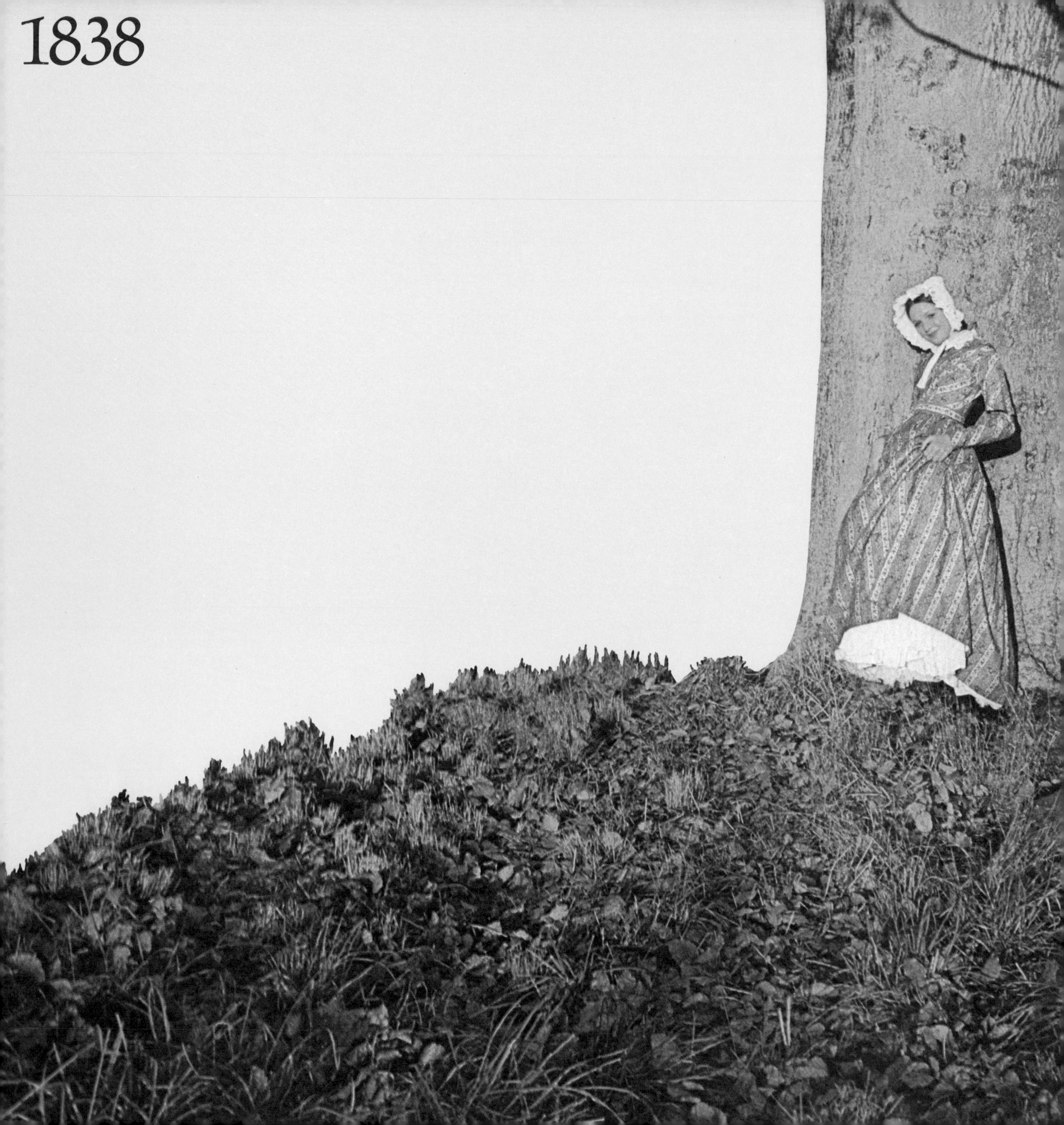

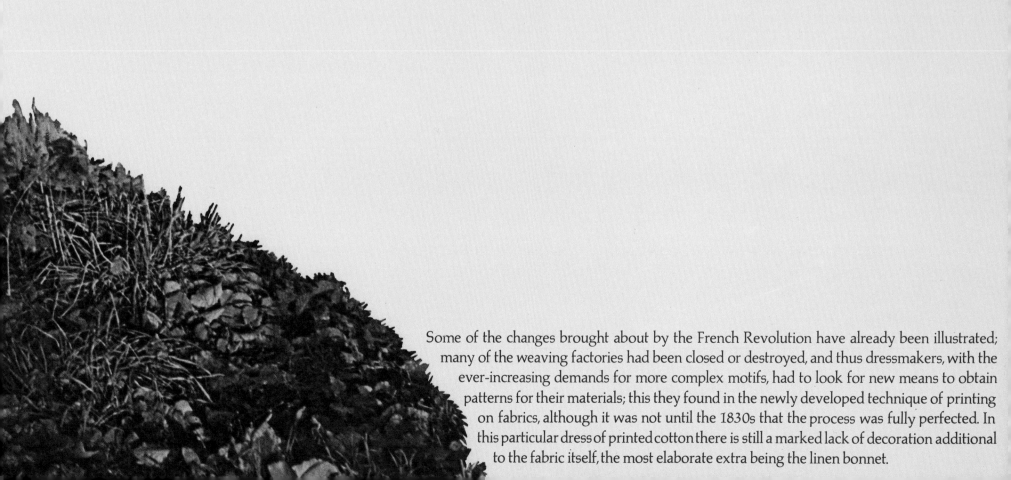

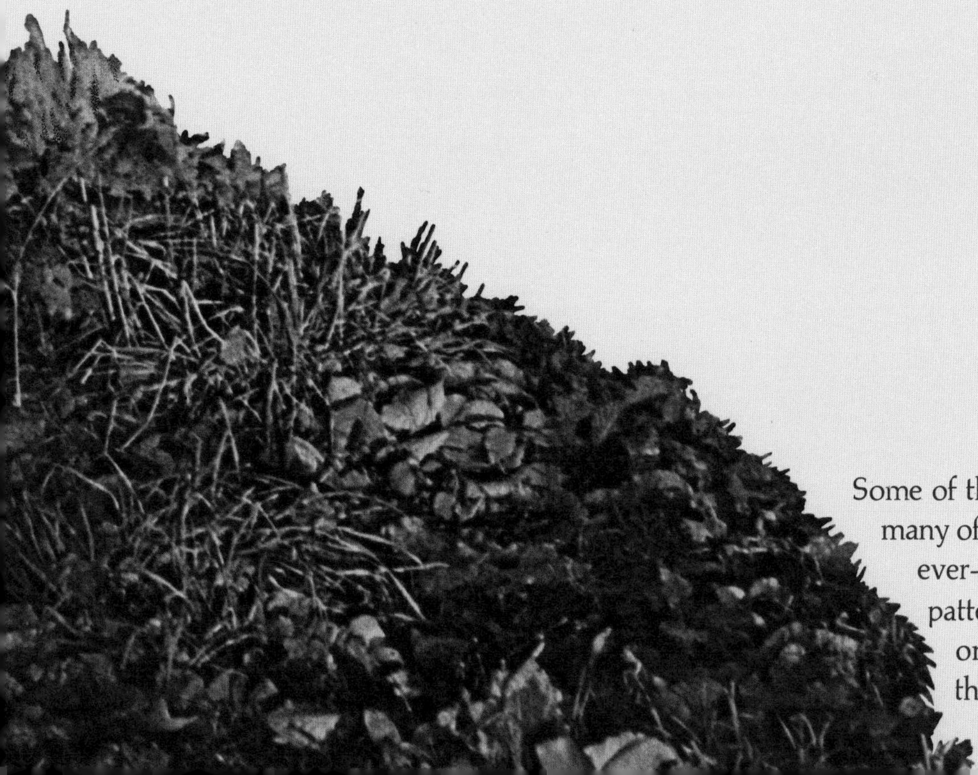

Some of the changes brought about by the French Revolution have already been illustrated; many of the weaving factories had been closed or destroyed, and thus dressmakers, with the ever-increasing demands for more complex motifs, had to look for new means to obtain patterns for their materials; this they found in the newly developed technique of printing on fabrics, although it was not until the 1830s that the process was fully perfected. In this particular dress of printed cotton there is still a marked lack of decoration additional to the fabric itself, the most elaborate extra being the linen bonnet.

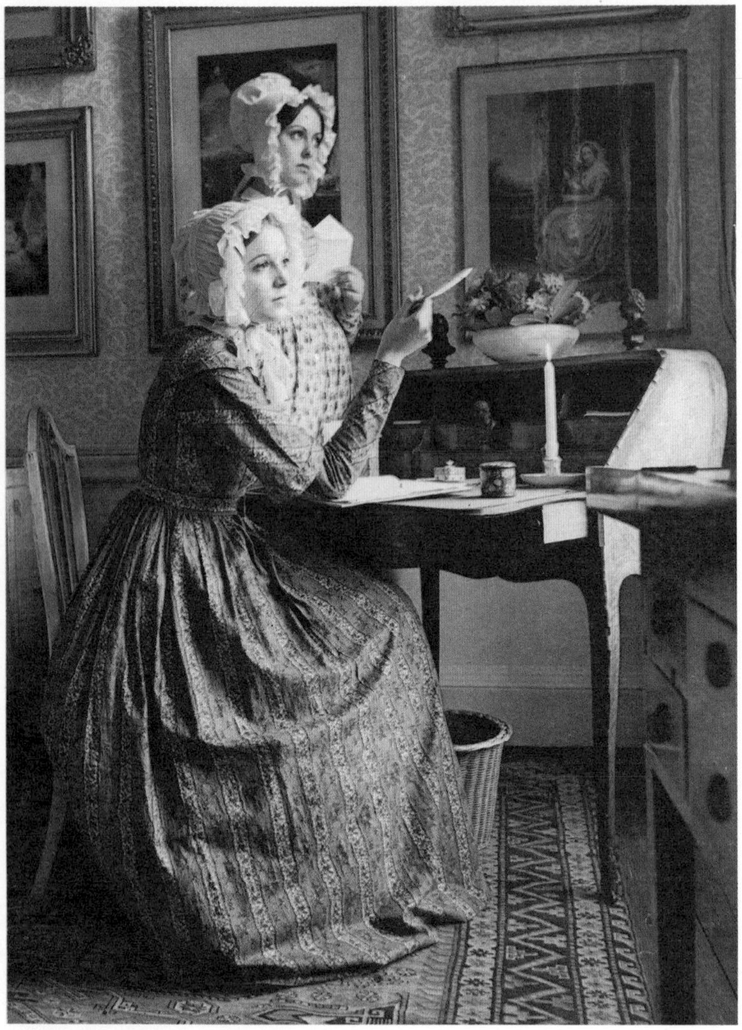

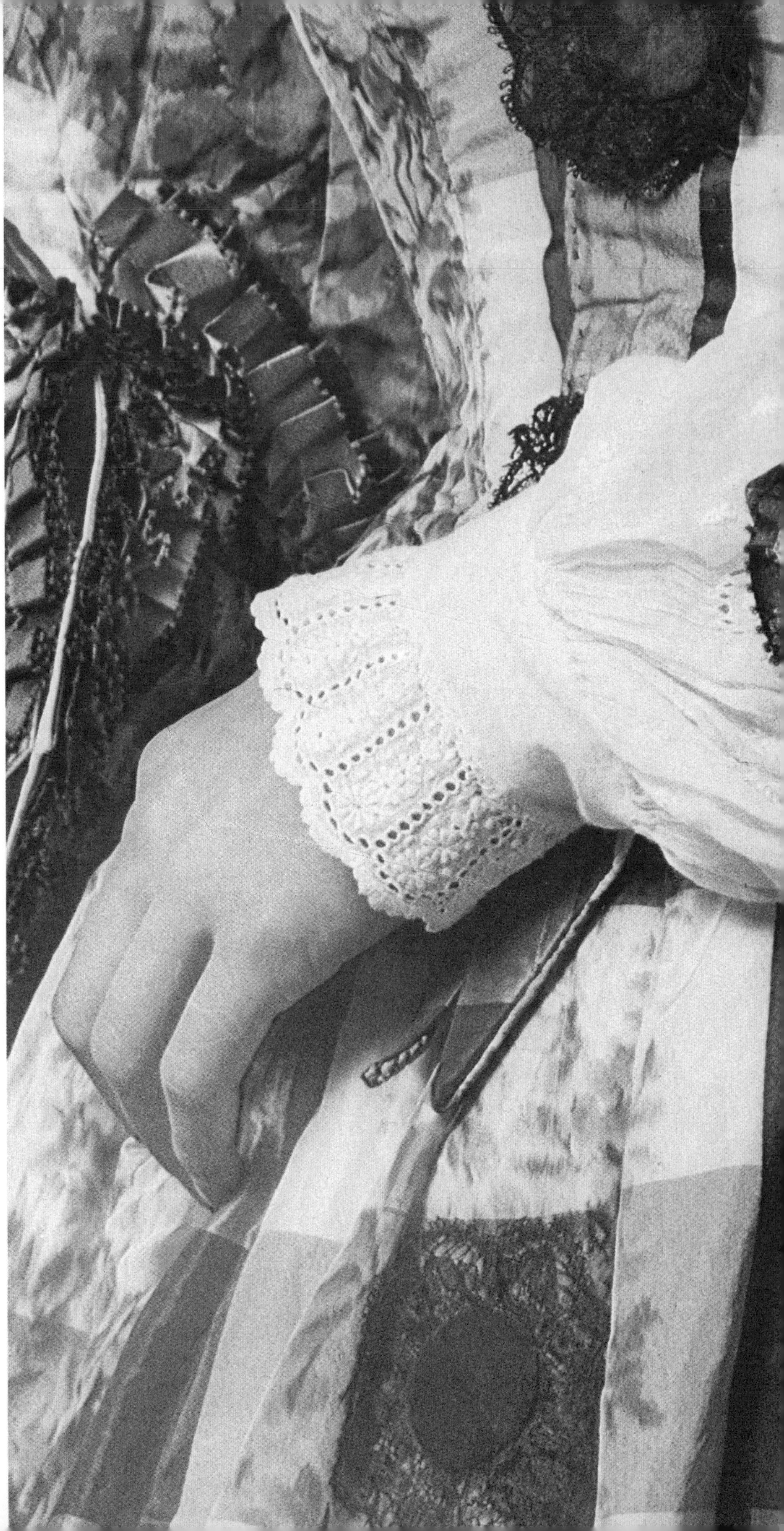

1838

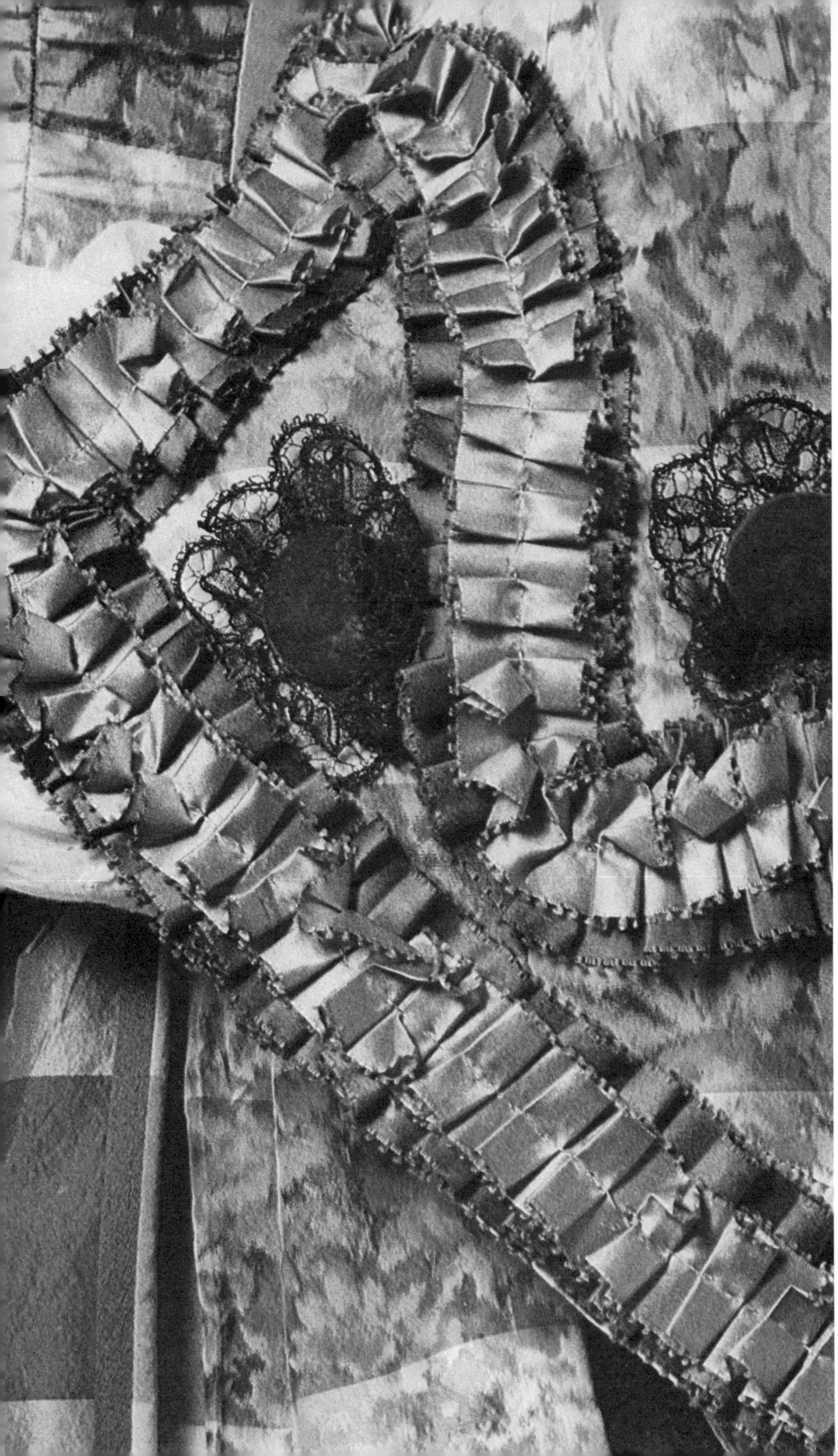

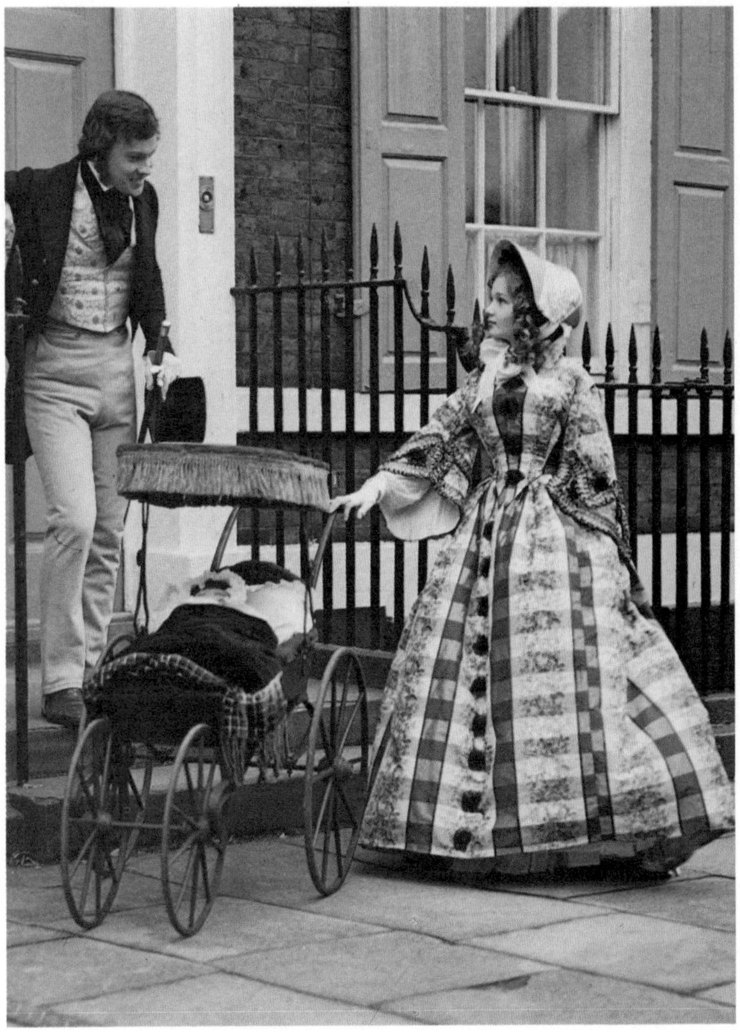

The printed silk trousseau dress of 1855 (this page) shows the re-emergence of more intricate decoration and forming: the brown velvet trimmings, black lace rosettes and hooped petticoats are all indicative of the style prevalent during Queen Victoria's reign. The man's suit is one worn by Samuel Wise at his wedding in Ripon in 1842, and includes the stays that accentuated the slim waist so fashionable at that time. (At the beginning of the 19th century, trousers had superseded knee breeches, and the top hat, in various forms, had become virtually the only headgear worn.)

1855

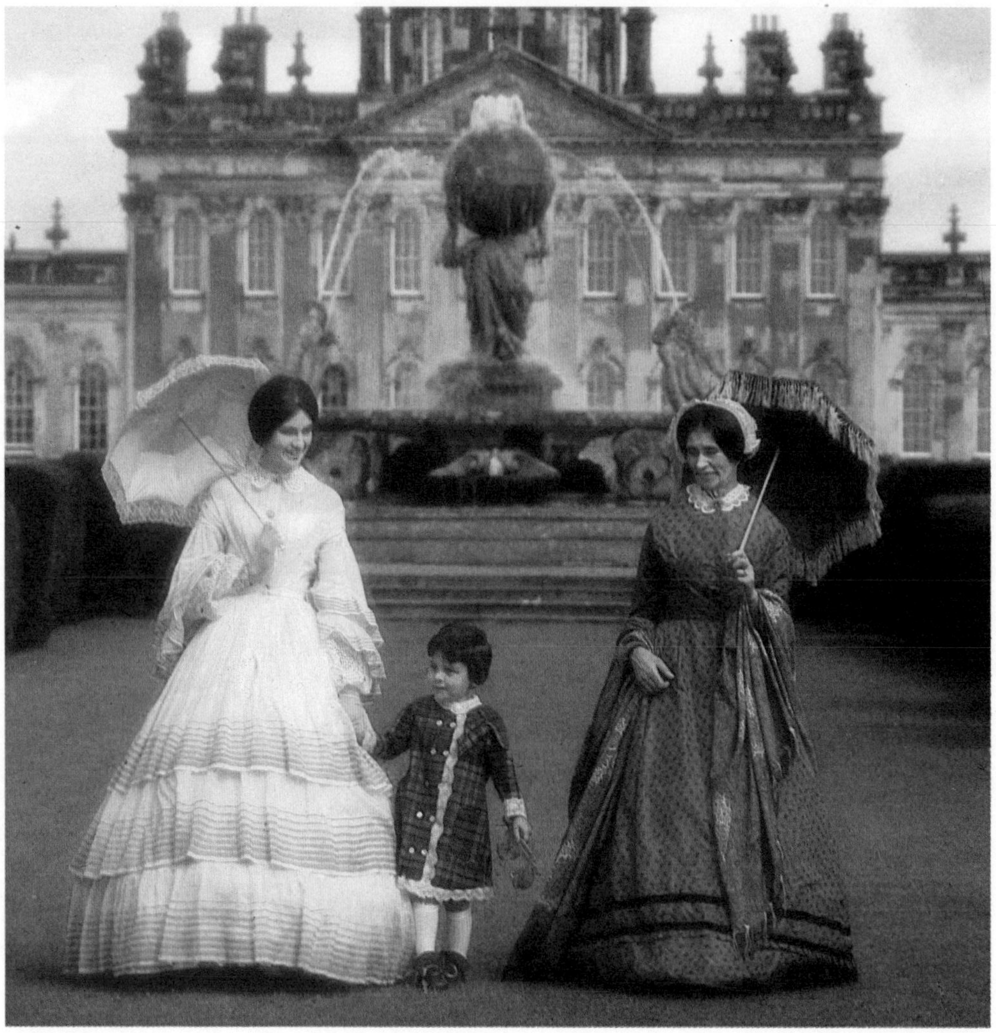

1855-1878

By the early 1860s the crinoline dress was the overriding fashion, often worn a few inches off the ground, displaying elegantly embroidered boots; those illustrated on this page are by Pinet, and were in fact made in about 1870. But these two day dresses, one of green printed silk, and the other white muslin with pale blue woven bands, mark the imminent departure of the crinoline from a lady's wardrobe. As the skirt billowed more and more in the rear, it was pulled up in a bunch, thus revealing the underskirt, and forming the basis of the bustle, which can be seen on the opposite page. The afternoon dress in blue and white muslin stripe of about 1868 is more restrained than the woven bustle dress in blue and cream silk, with its porcelain buttons, of 1878. (The detail of this dress can be seen above right and on the cover.)

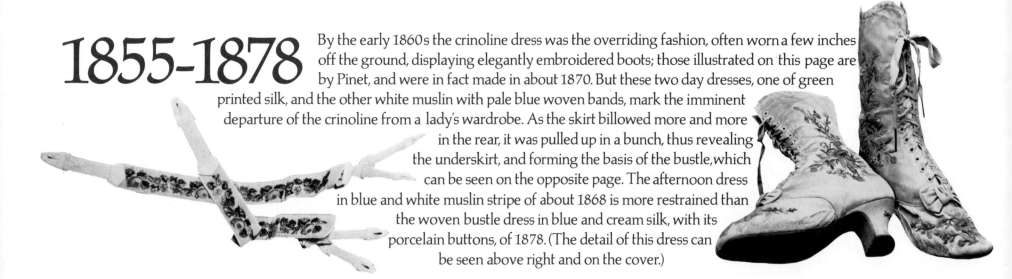

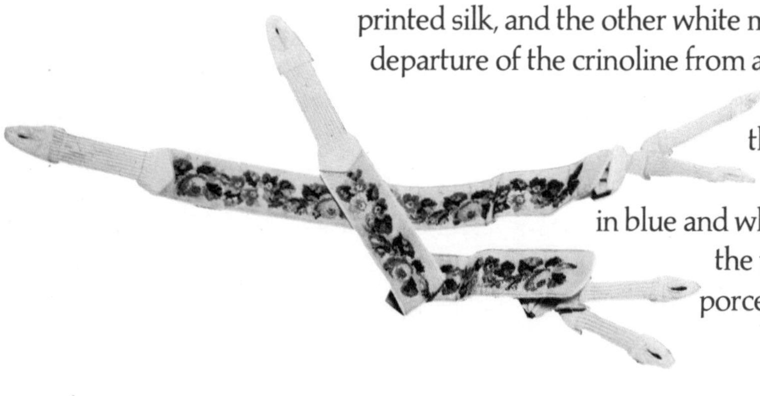

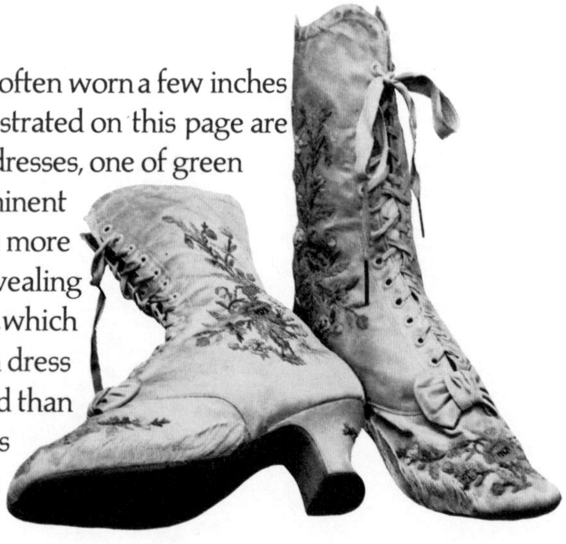

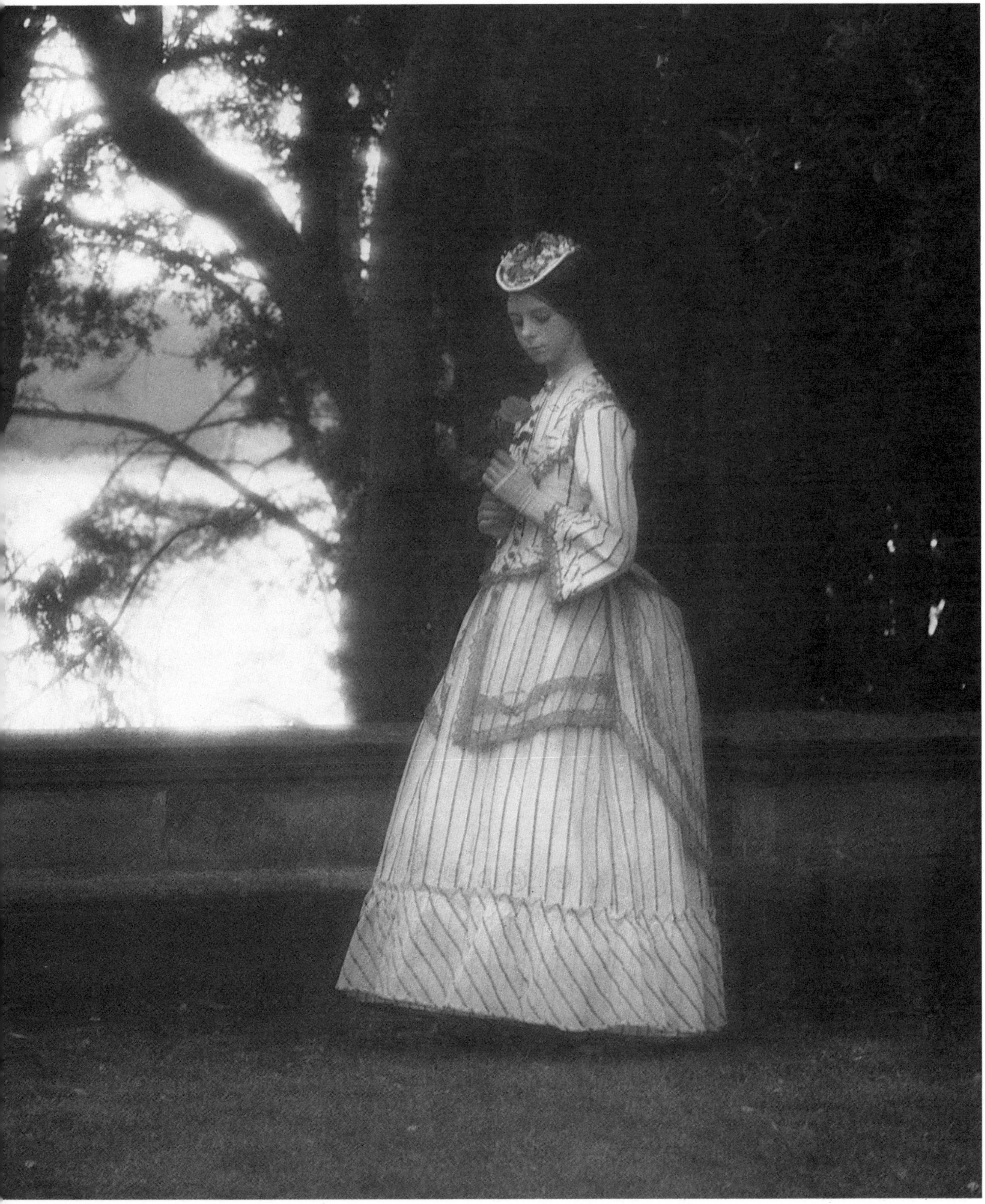
 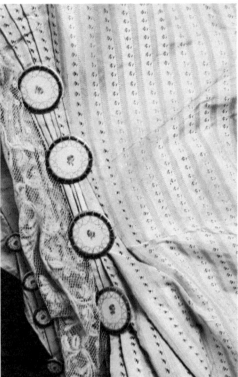
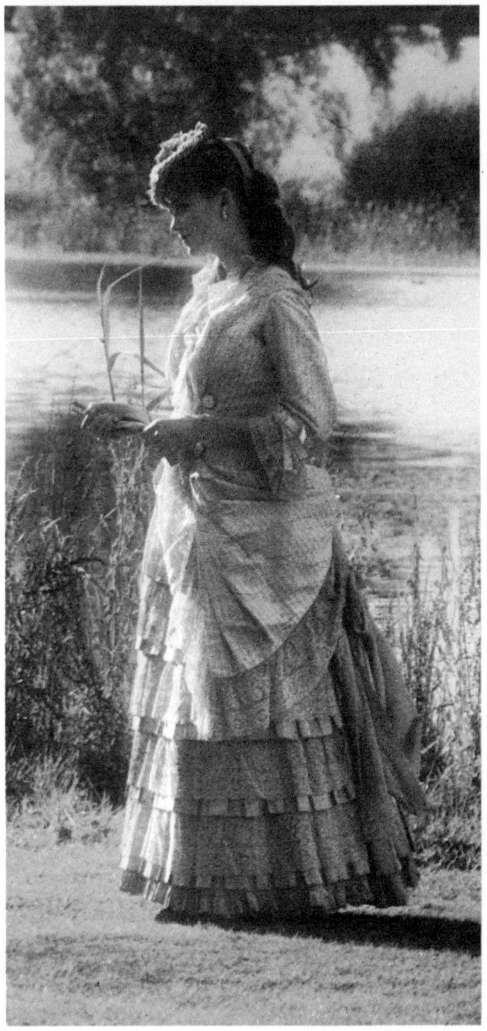

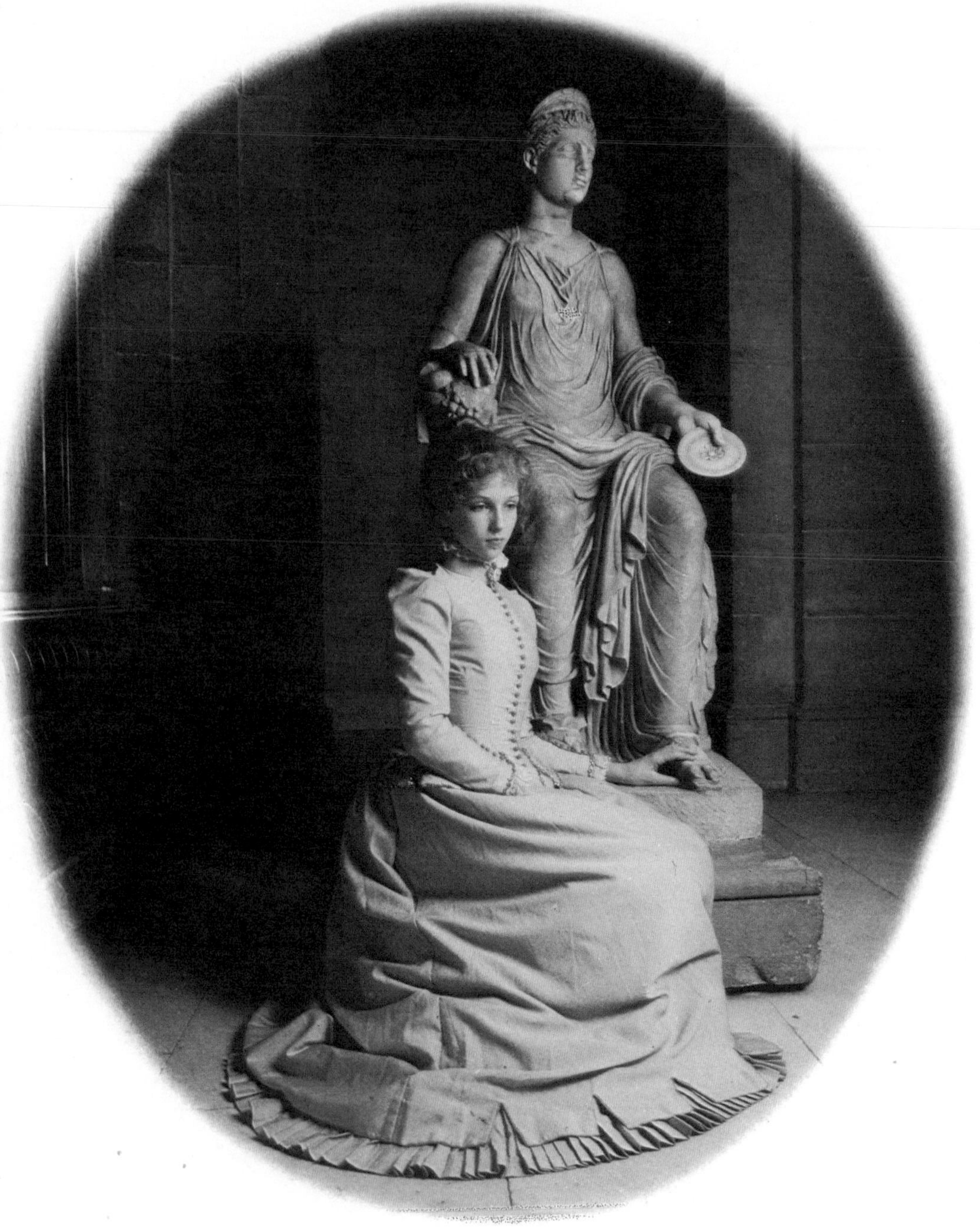

1890 The public morality of Victorian society lent itself to a sombre note in dress, particularly in younger people, as is evident in this young lady's fine wool dress of 1890, trimmed with cut steel.

1900 The 1900 Court presentation dress of satin embroidered with pearls presents a more elegant figure, which points towards the Edwardian flamboyance that is soon to show itself.

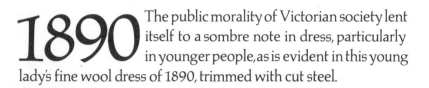

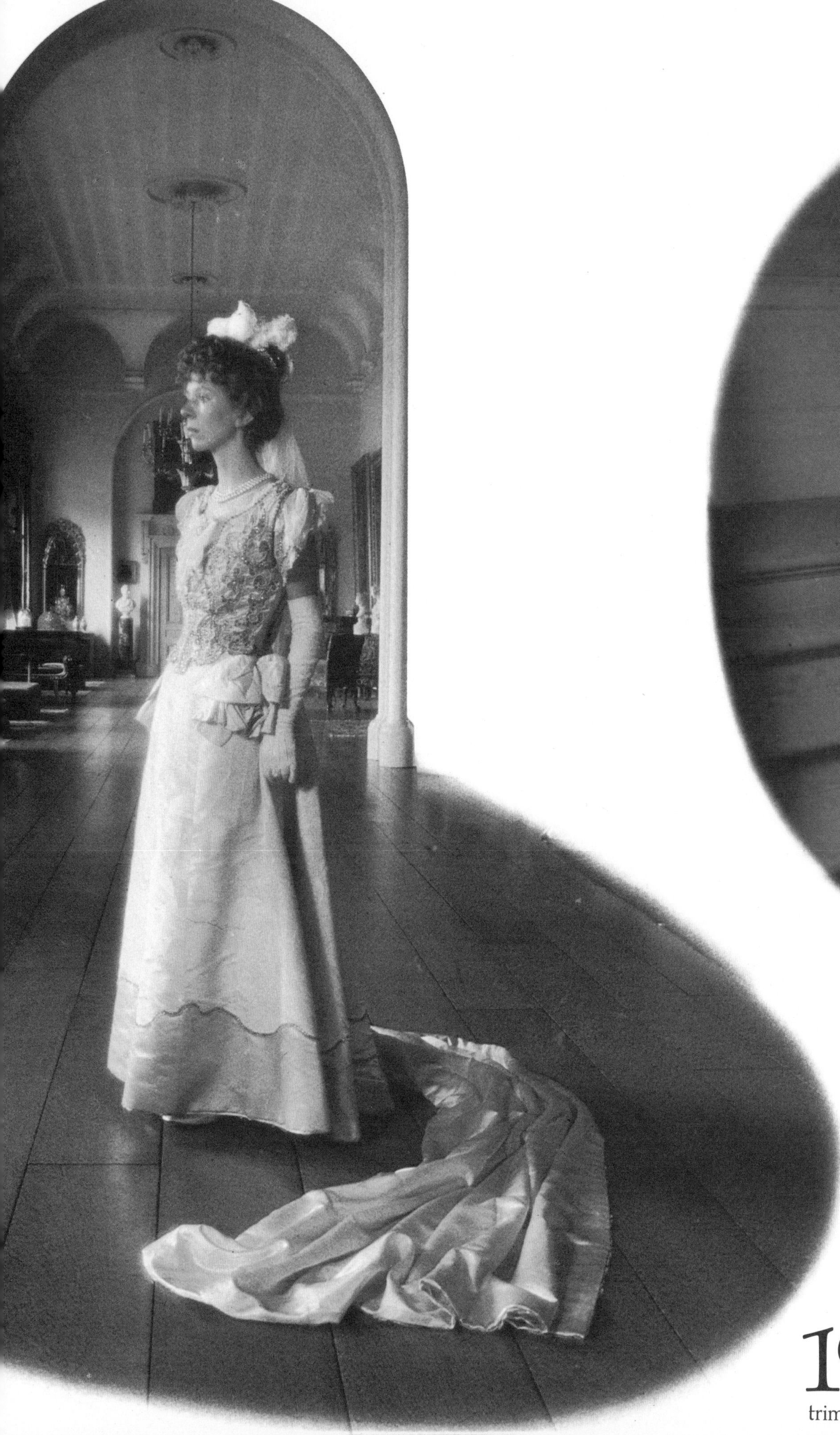

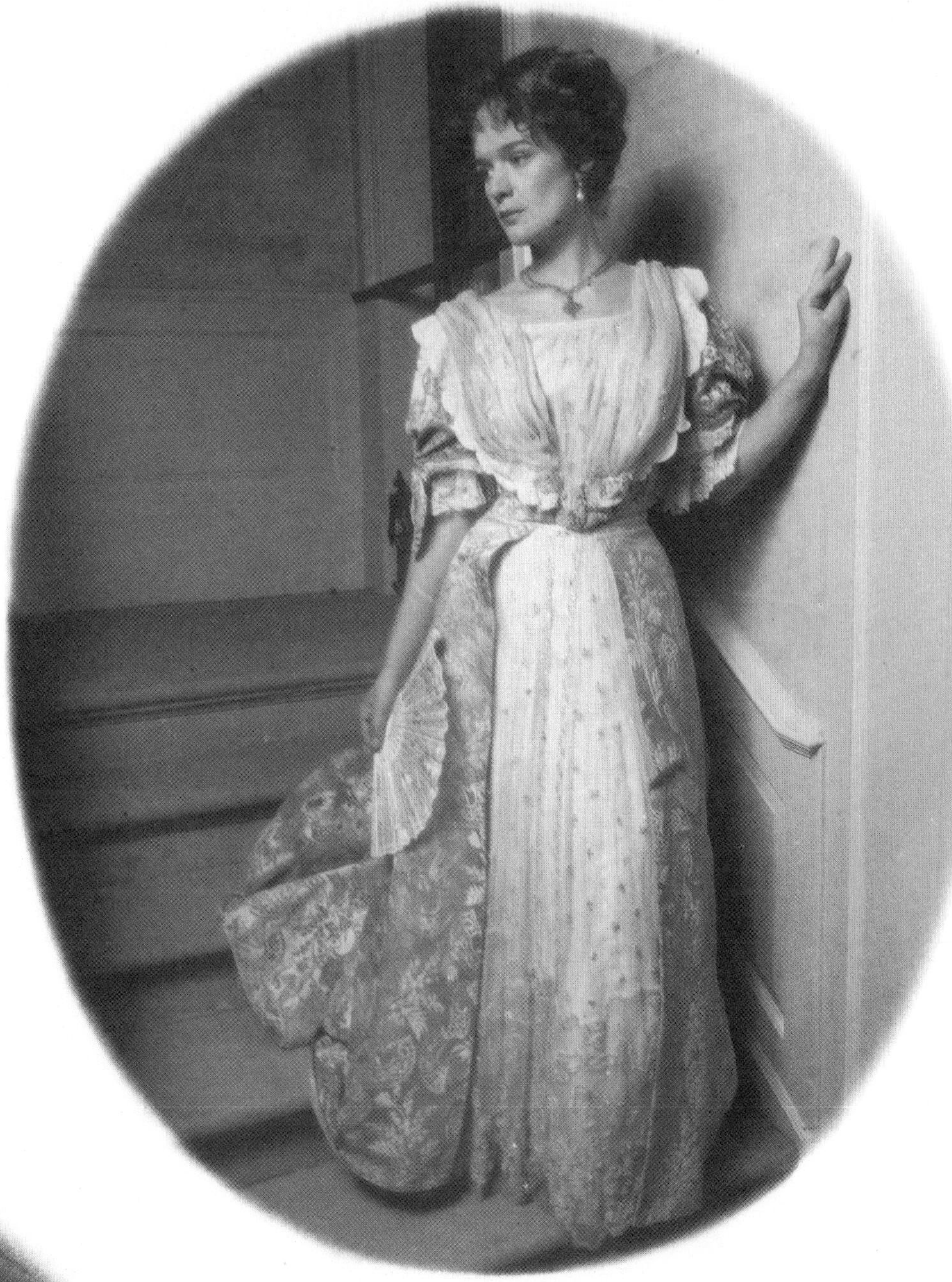

1904

This mauve cut velvet gown, worn in about 1904, projects a more voluptuous figure, with its beaded chiffon petticoats and trimmings; the tiny waist accentuates the bust and hips.

1907

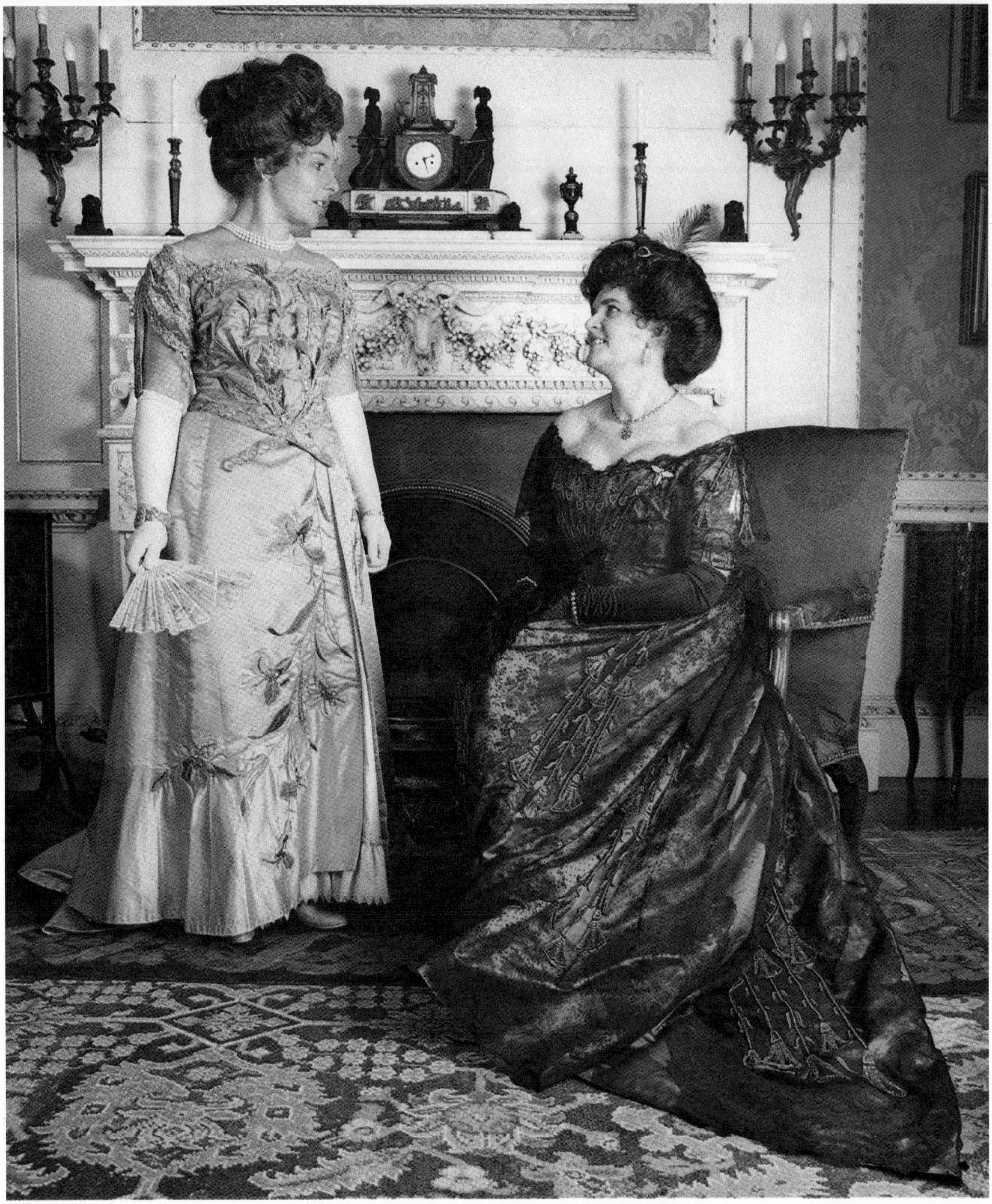

There is little restraint in the decoration of this yellow satin evening dress with its elaborate silver lace and chenille embroidery, or the blue brocade (by Worth), festooned in black lace and beadwork. Both of these are typical of their date, with low, wide neck lines, short sleeves and sweeping hems, worn with long gloves forever flickering the fan.

The lady descending from the landau carriage in a 1910 day dress of nuns' veiling and cotton lace is dressed quietly by comparison with many of her contemporaries, while the man's flamboyance is shown only in the buttonhole, the waistcoat, the spats and the braiding on his morning coat – light hearted decoration on basically restrained dress.

1910

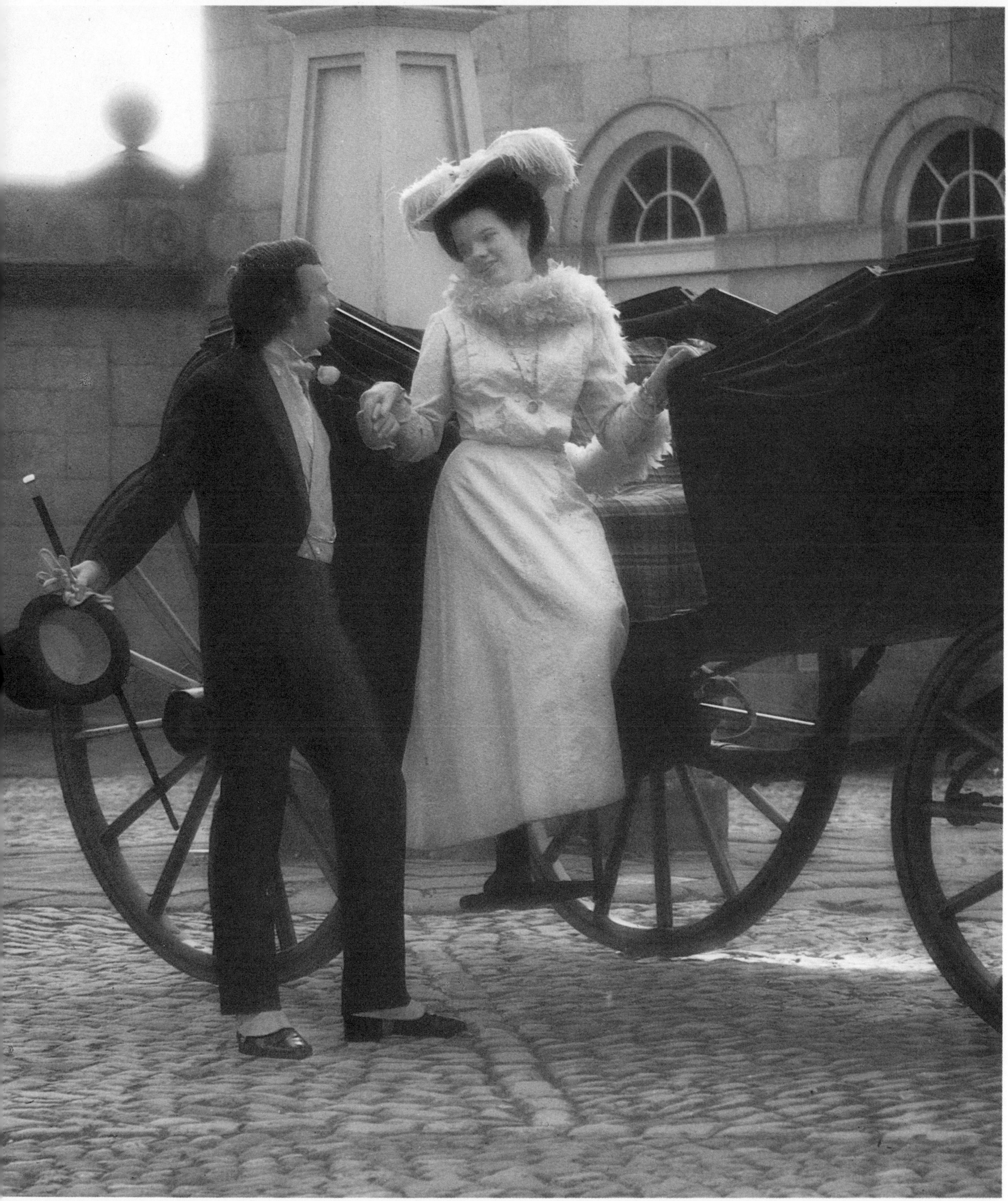

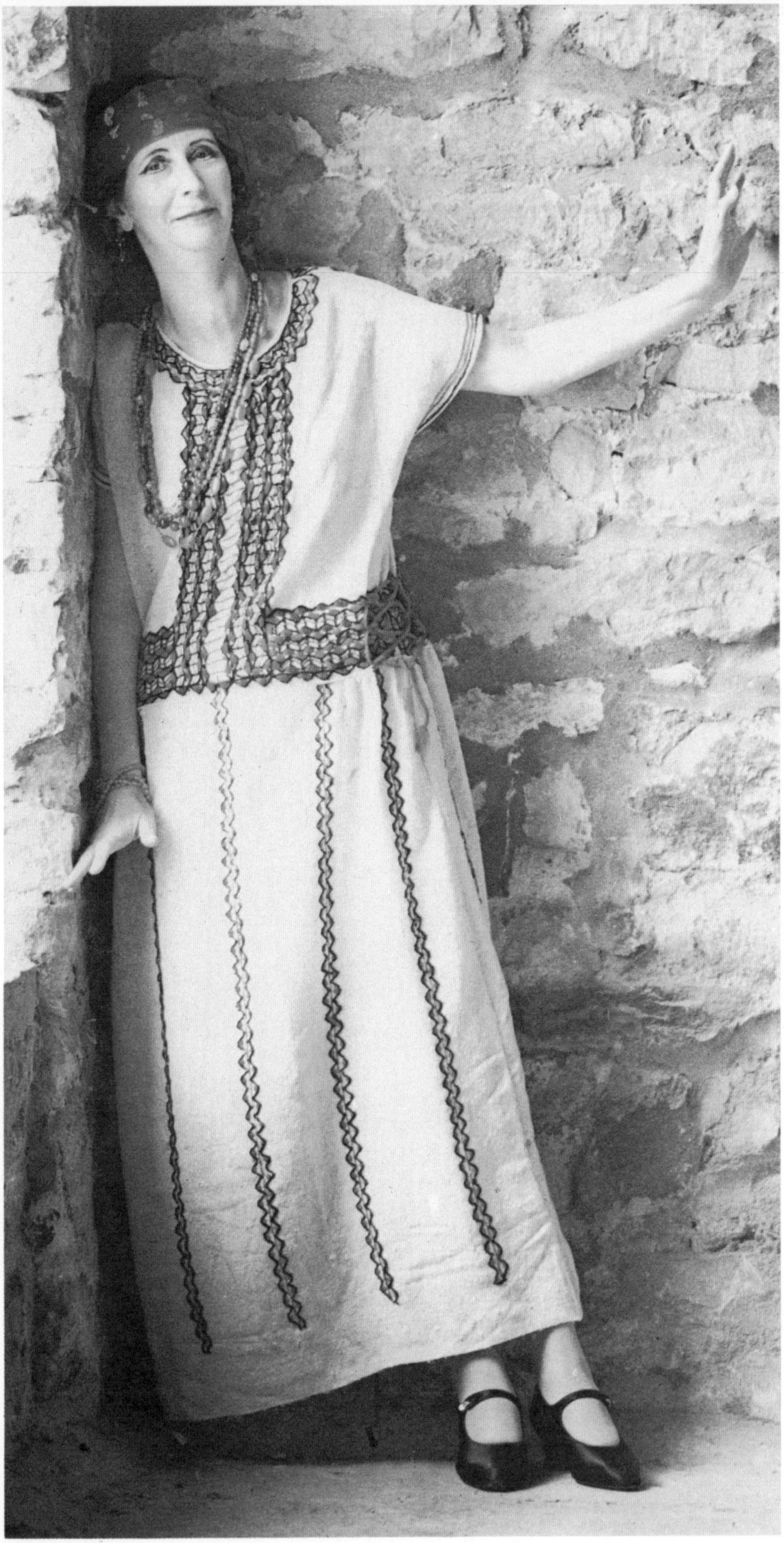

Reflected in this loosely woven cotton dress of 1920 are hints of ballet design, of "peasant" dress, and of exotic Eastern influence.

1920

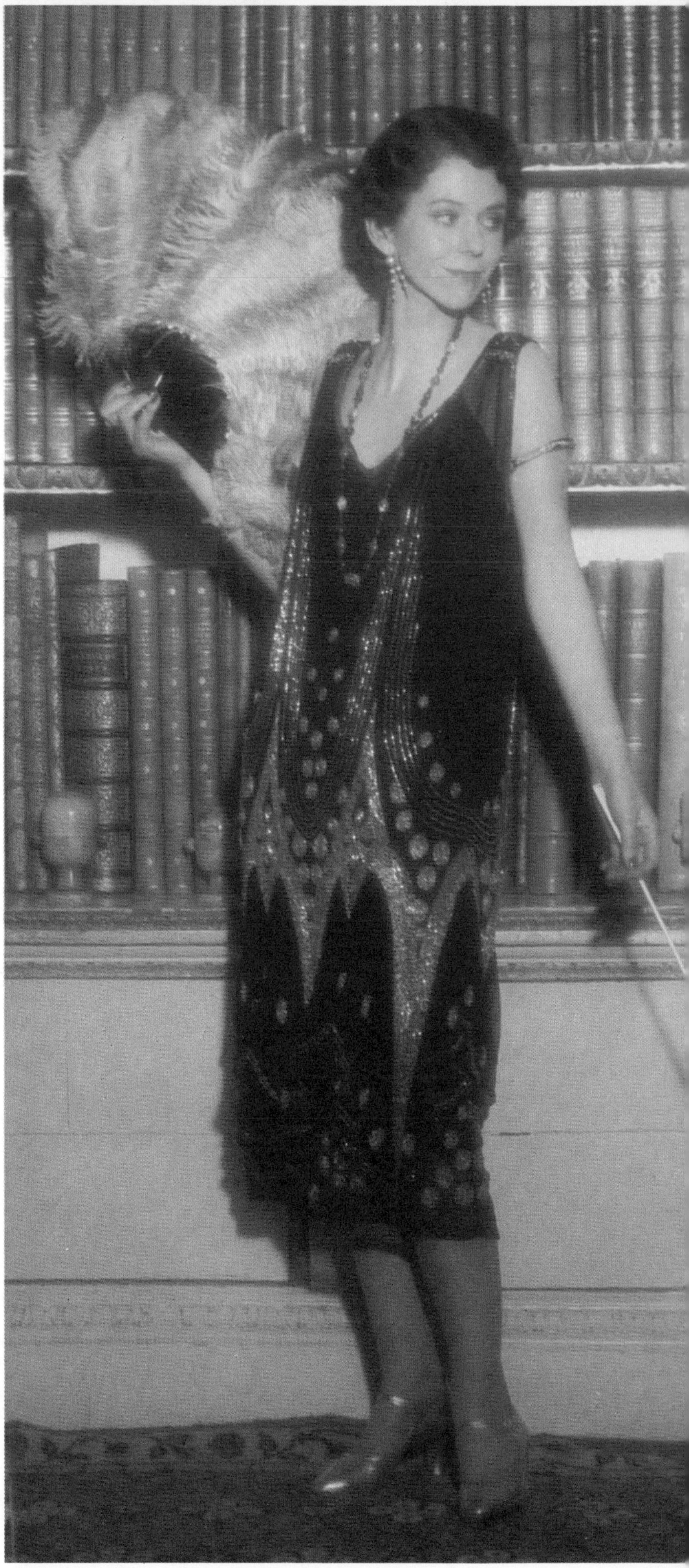

This 1924 flapper evening dress in black with glass beadwork swings loose from the shoulder, showing parts of the body never previously exposed, and portraying a casual attitude never previously experienc

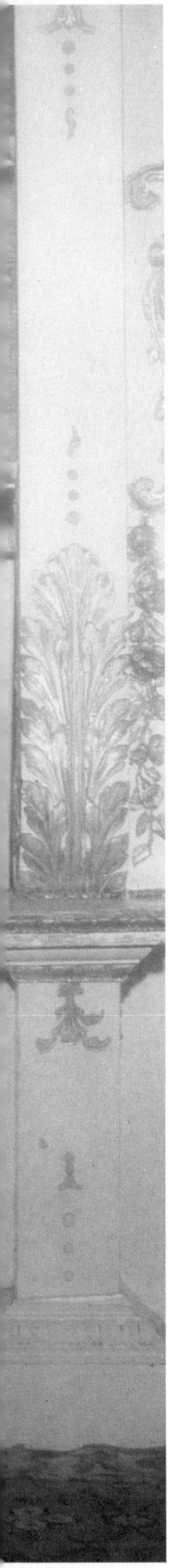

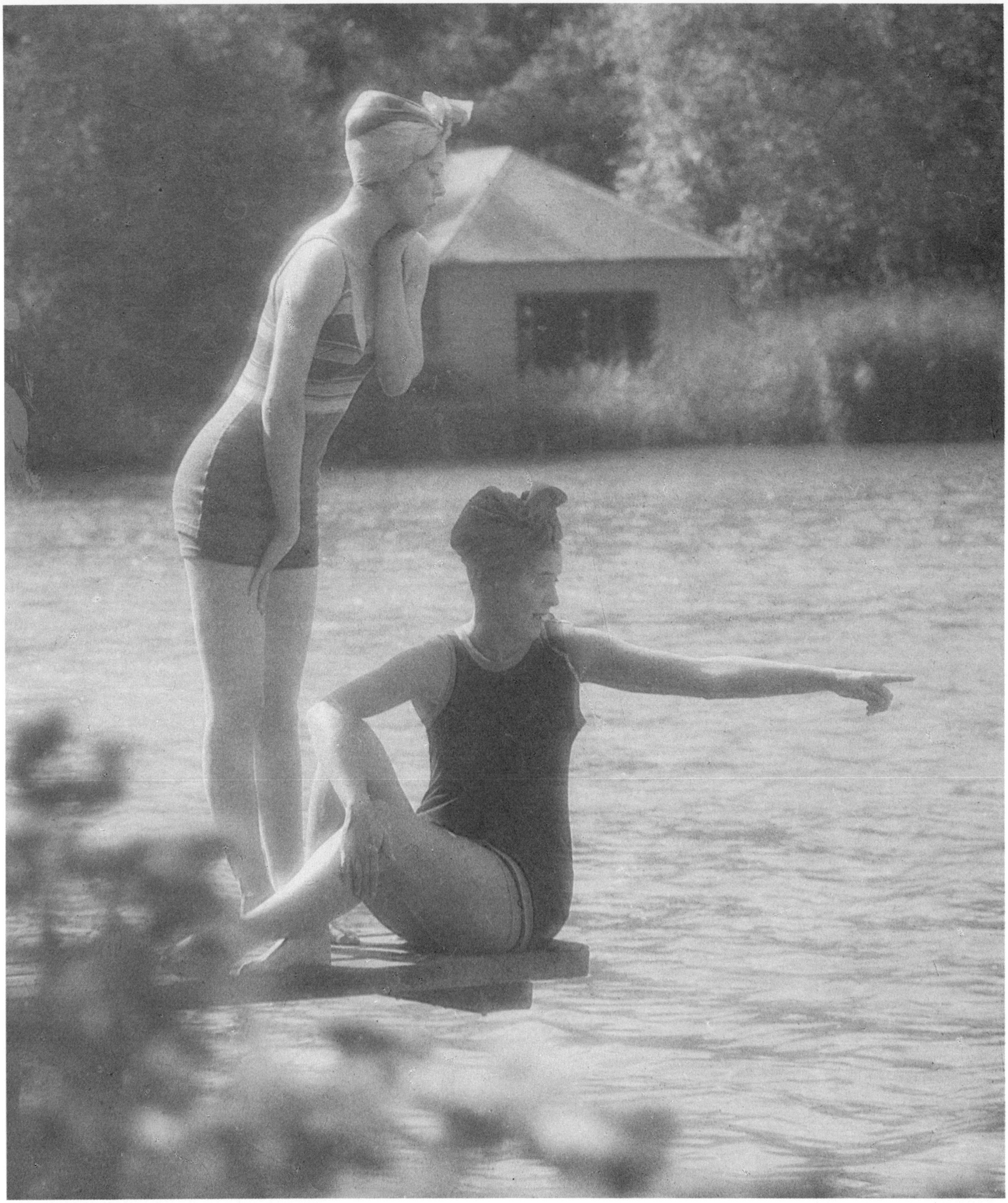

1924

The close of the First War had seen great changes in fashion, paralleling the rigorous social changes of the period. The bathing dresses shown here and on the following pages are a further illustration of the reckless abandoning of formalities, with their unfamiliar displays of naked arms and legs.

1927

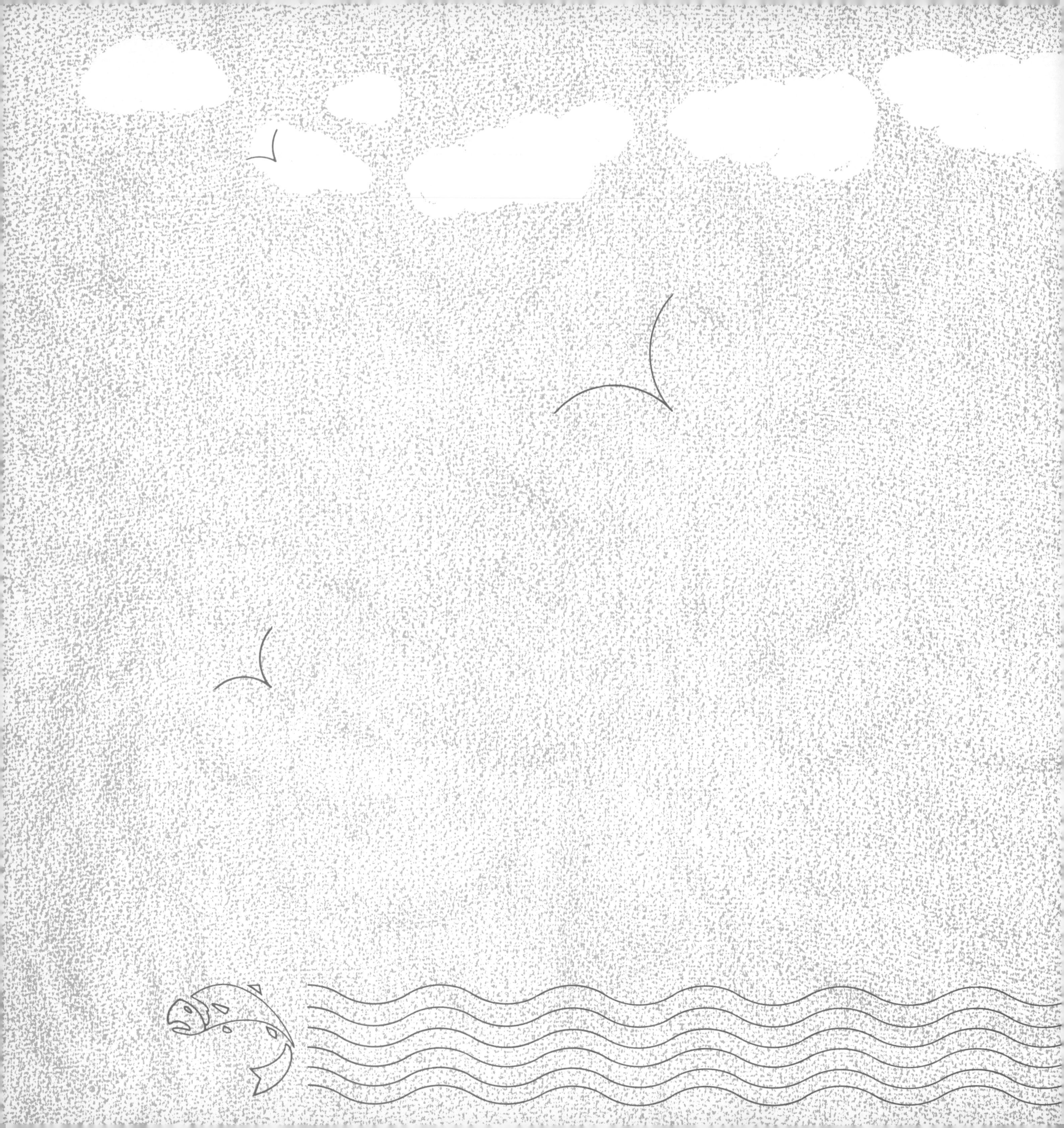

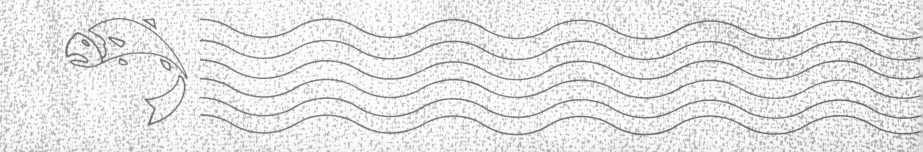

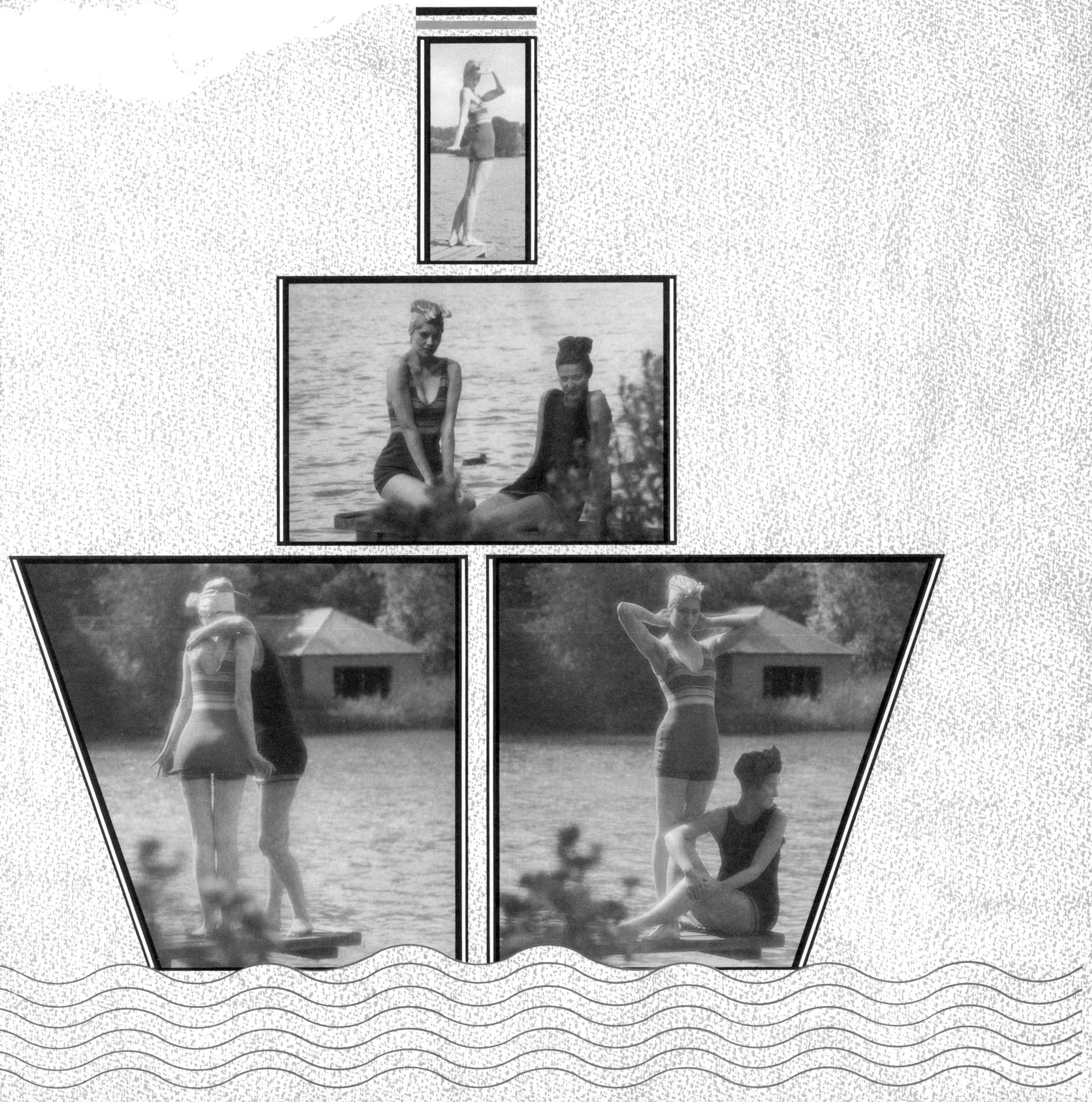

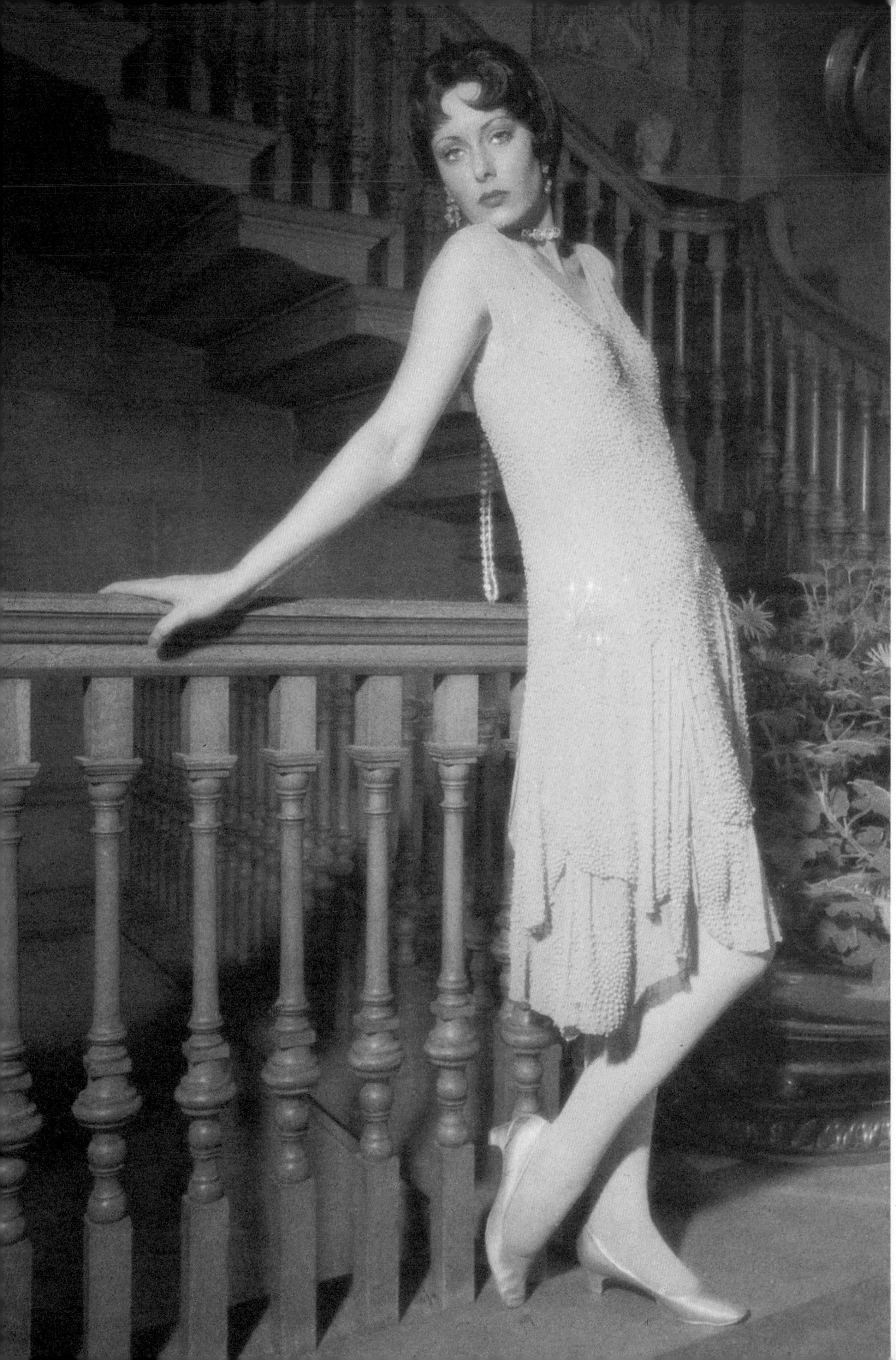

1927 The near-shapelessness of the flapper had been replaced now by the clinging looks of this pink chiffon evening dress, encrusted from neck to hem in coral beads, and decorated with crystal medallions.

Shown on the right is a 1932 gold lace evening dress, studded with diamanté, over which is worn a French gold lamé bridge coat, embroidered with diamanté and pearls.

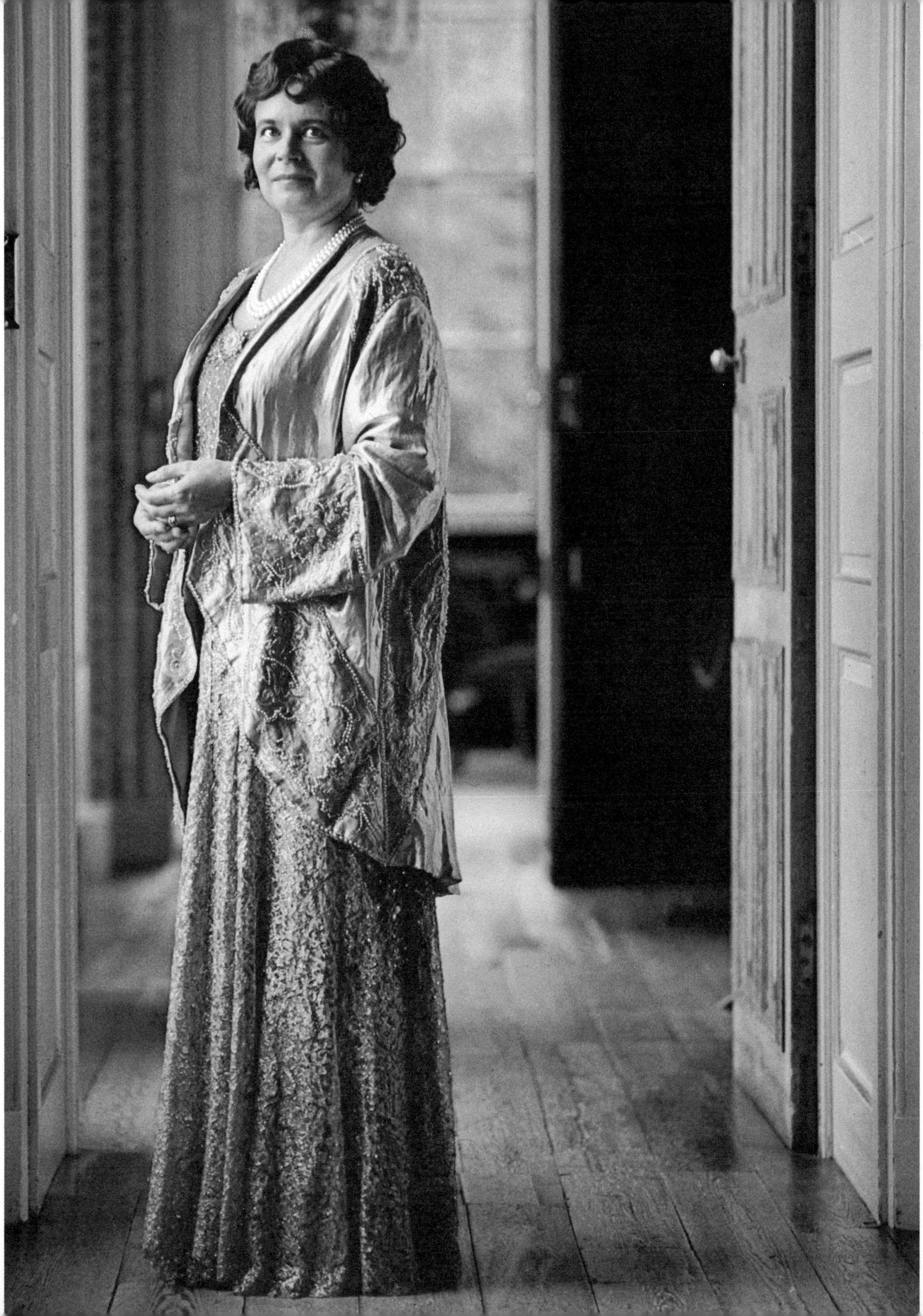

1932

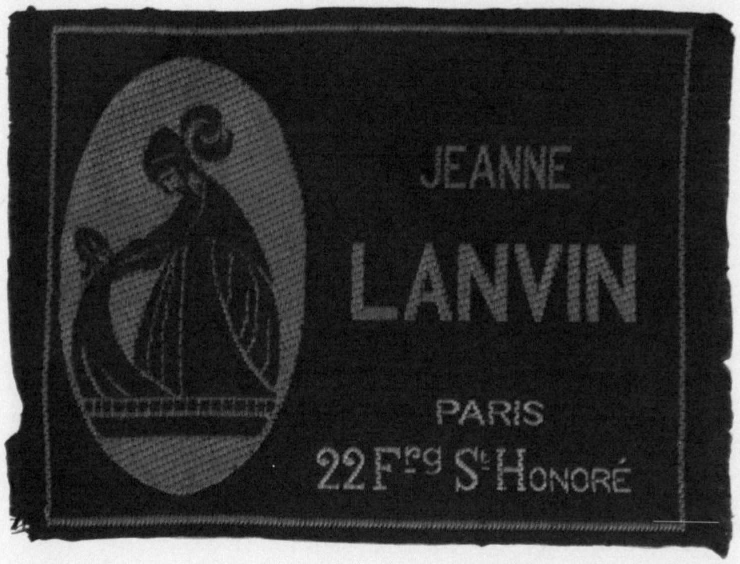

1935 Both the orange velvet evening coat with its red fox fur collar, shown on this page, and the evening dress of black ciré ribbon on net (overleaf) were made by Lanvin in 1935; by this date, the focus of attention was once more on slim waists, graceful curves and long, elegant figures.

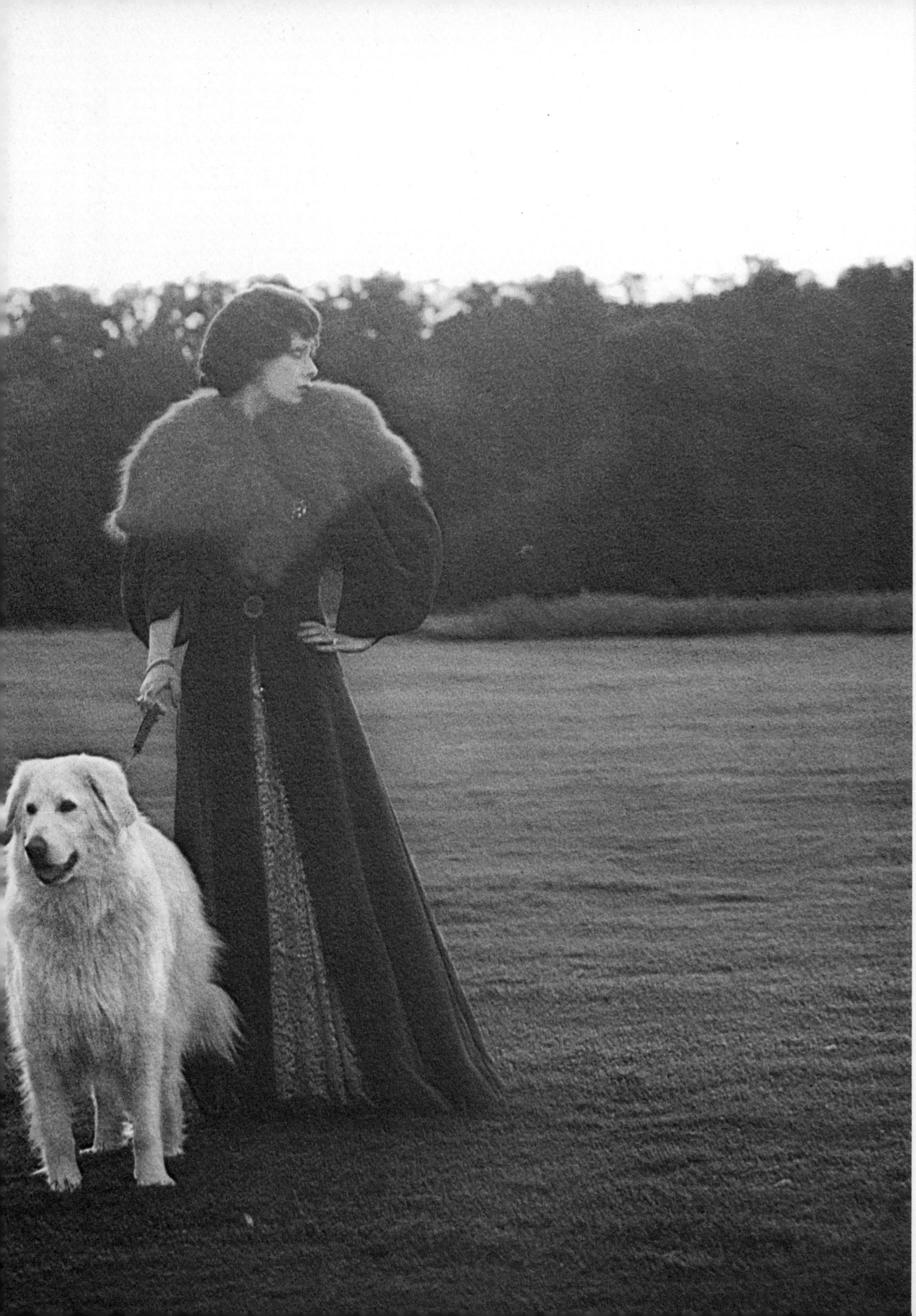

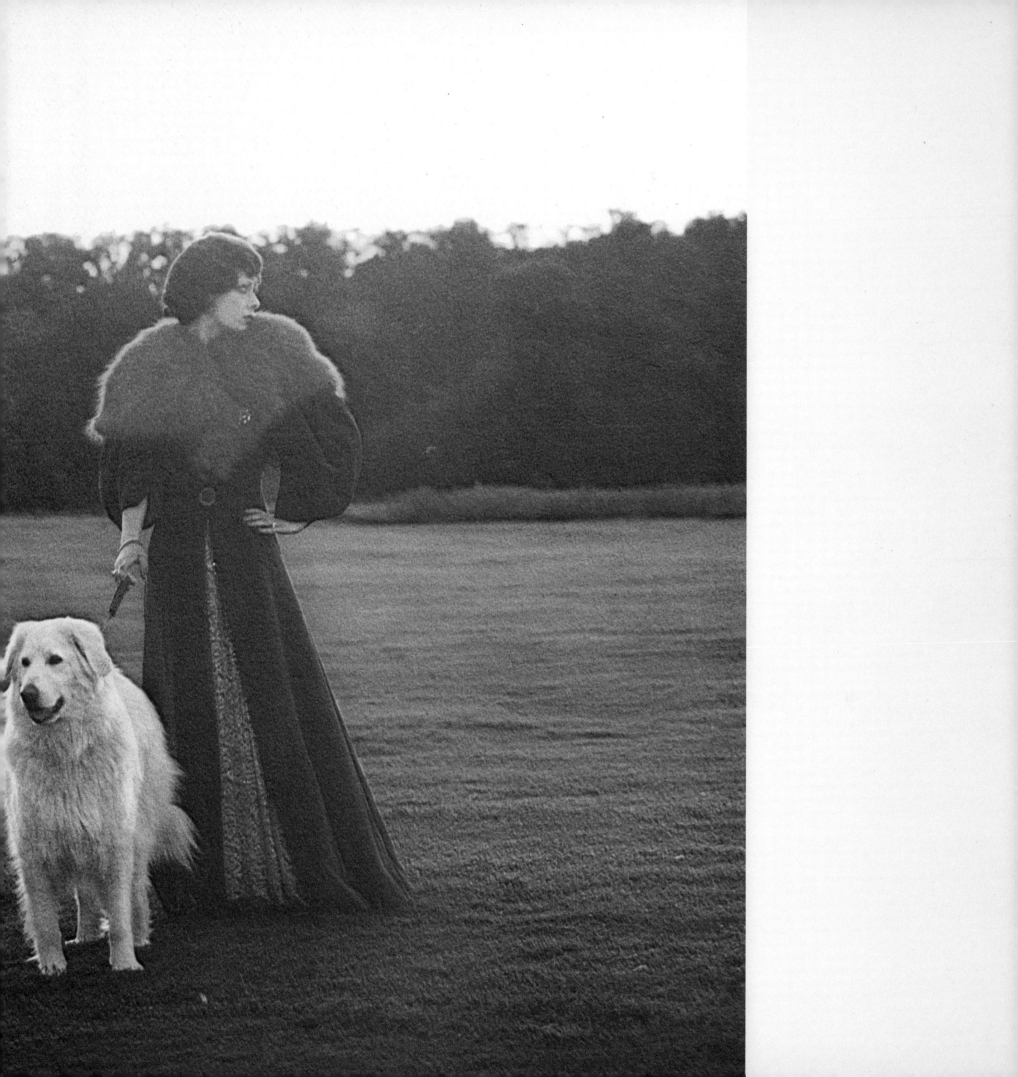

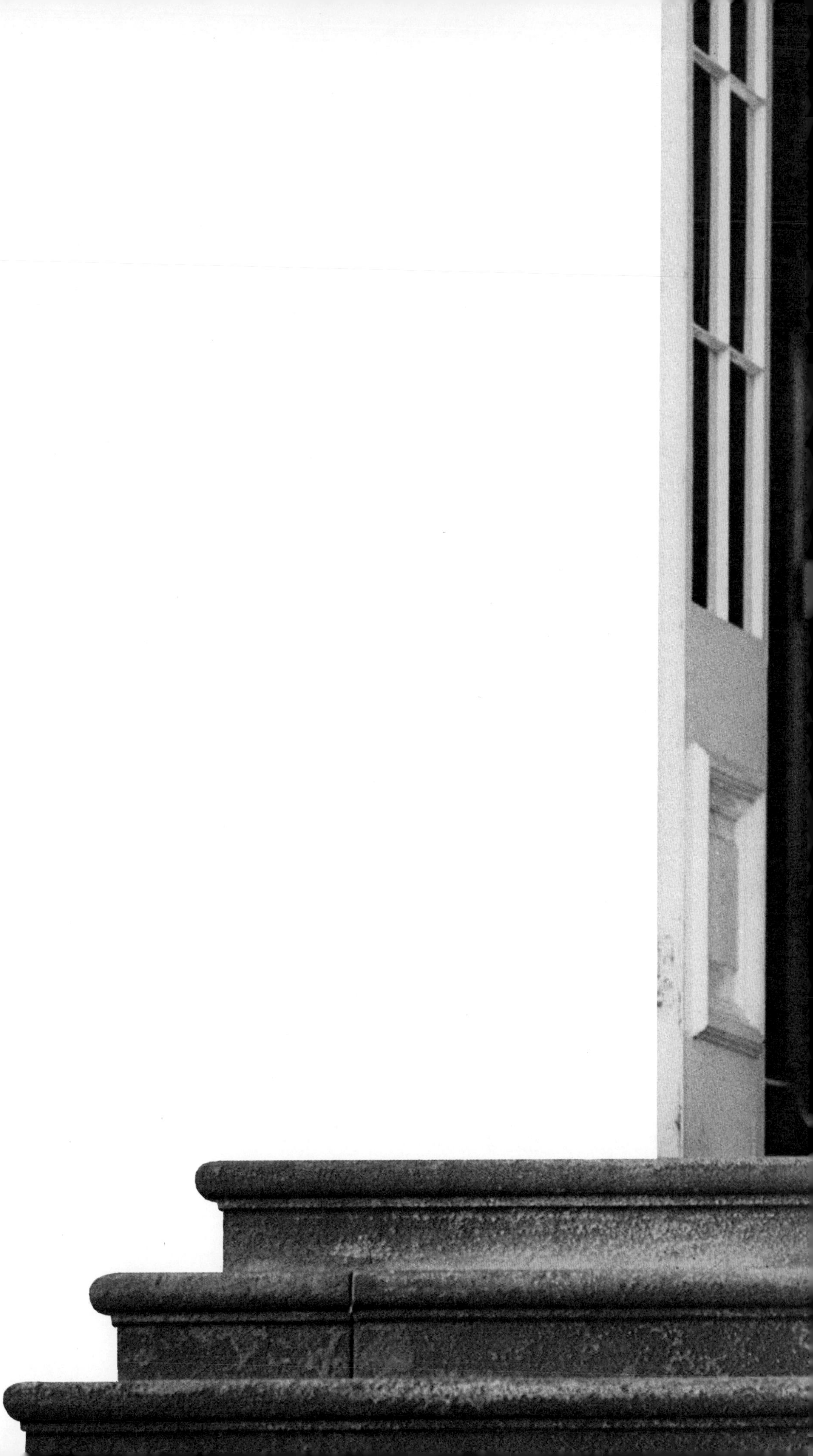

1935

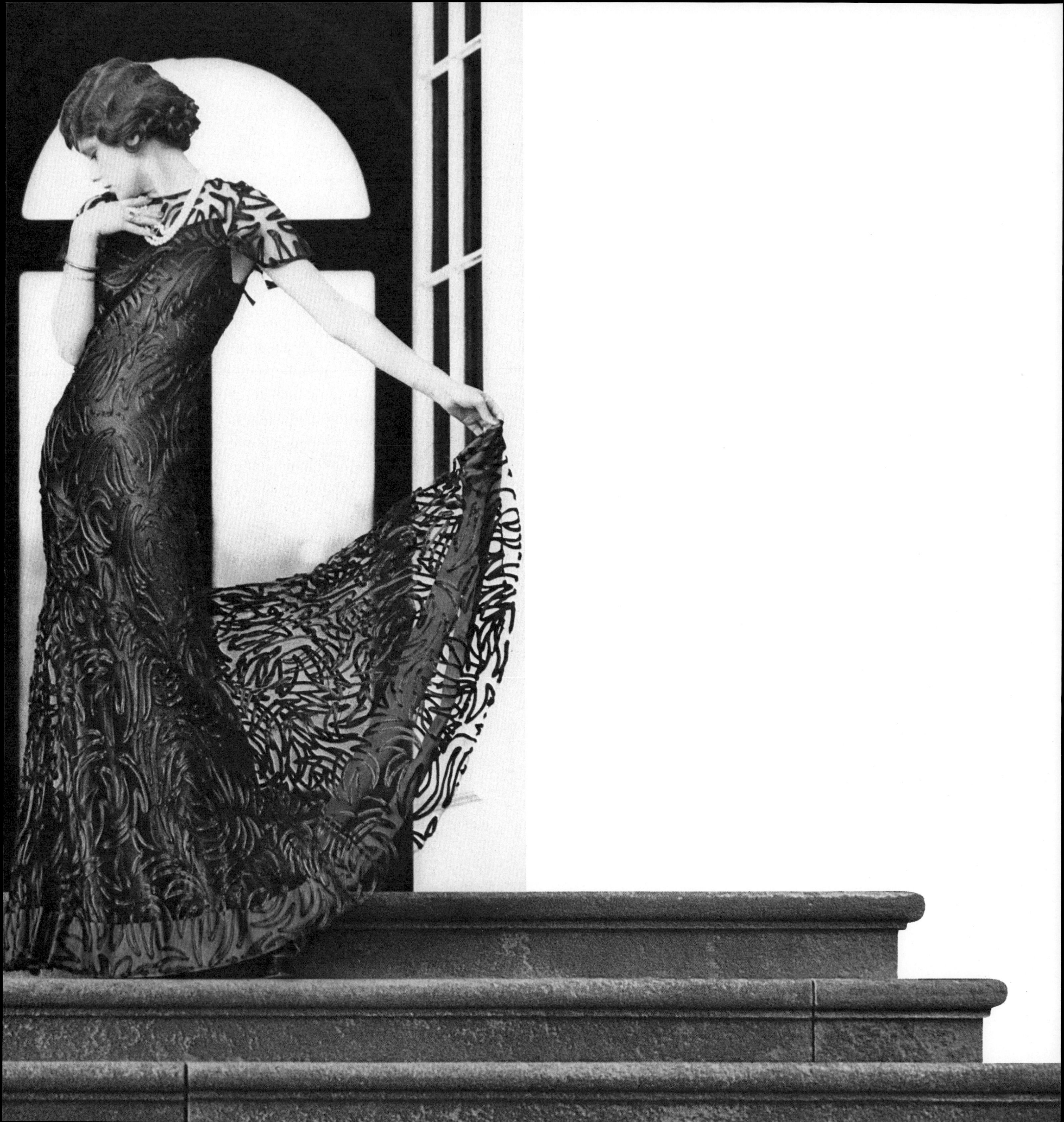

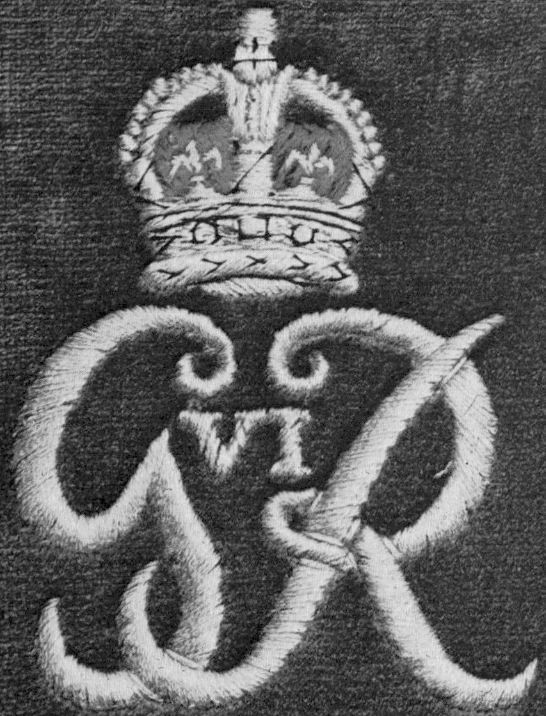

1937 The robes worn by a peer of the realm at a coronation are unique to that occasion; for example, completely different robes are worn at the opening of Parliament. Those shown on this page were worn by Susanna, Duchess of Grafton at the 1937 Coronation, and by the Duchess of Northumberland at the 1953 Coronation. They are made of velvet and edged with ermine. (It is interesting to note that while the tiara is worn throughout the service, peers and peeresses do not don their coronets until the very moment the monarch is crowned).

In the centre is the uniform of the Vice-Chamberlain of HM household; stitched to the back of his tail coat is a golden key. The page is dressed in the livery colours of the Duke of Norfolk, as worn at the Coronation of George VI.

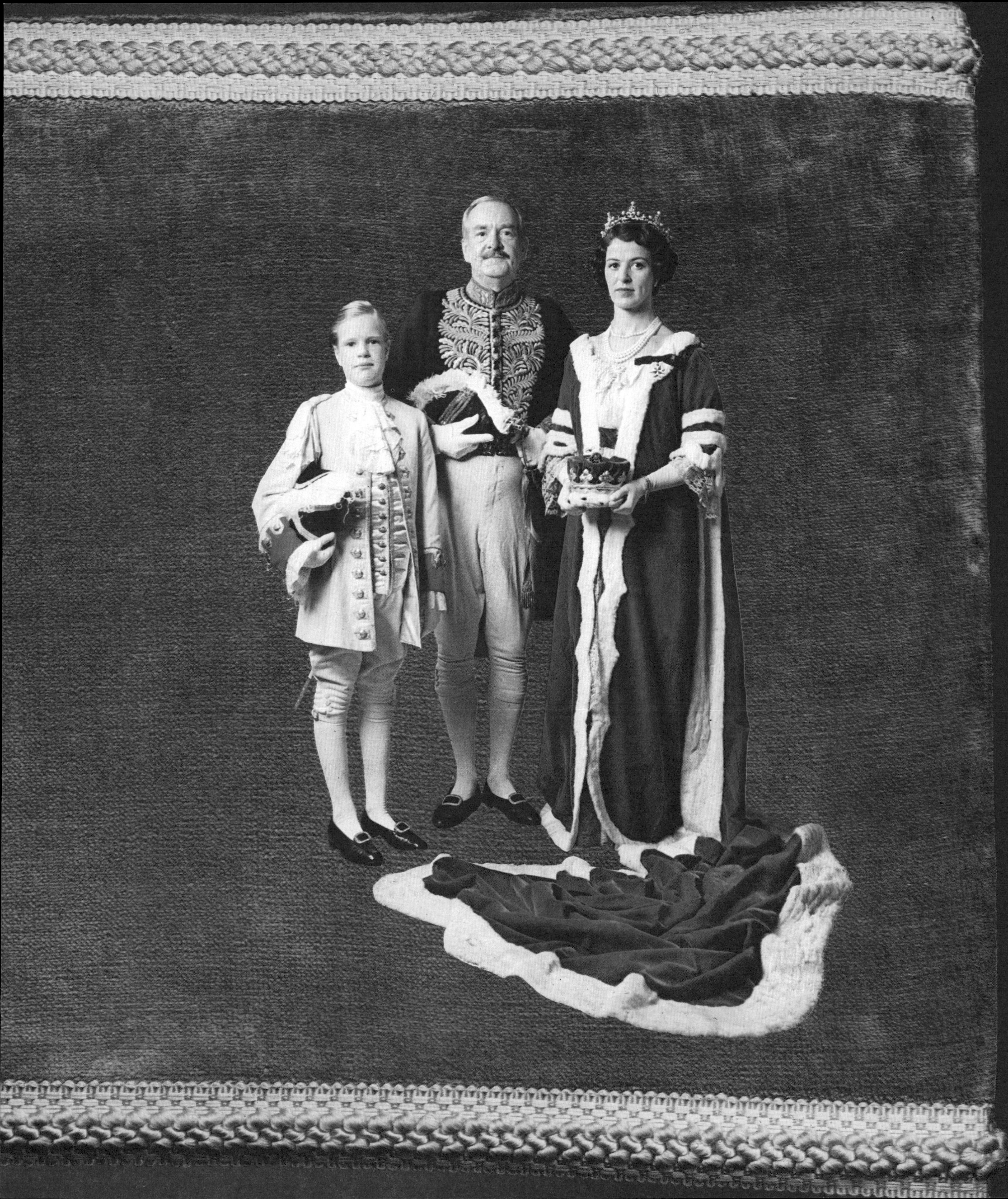

1947

By 1947, wartime austerity and rationing still held fashion well within the bounds of utility; but in the spring all this was overturned when Christian Dior unveiled his "new look," with its extravagant use of rich fabrics, the guepière waist, small shoulders, padded hips and long, full skirts. This was taken up immediately by every fashion-house, and the dress illustrated here is by Worth.

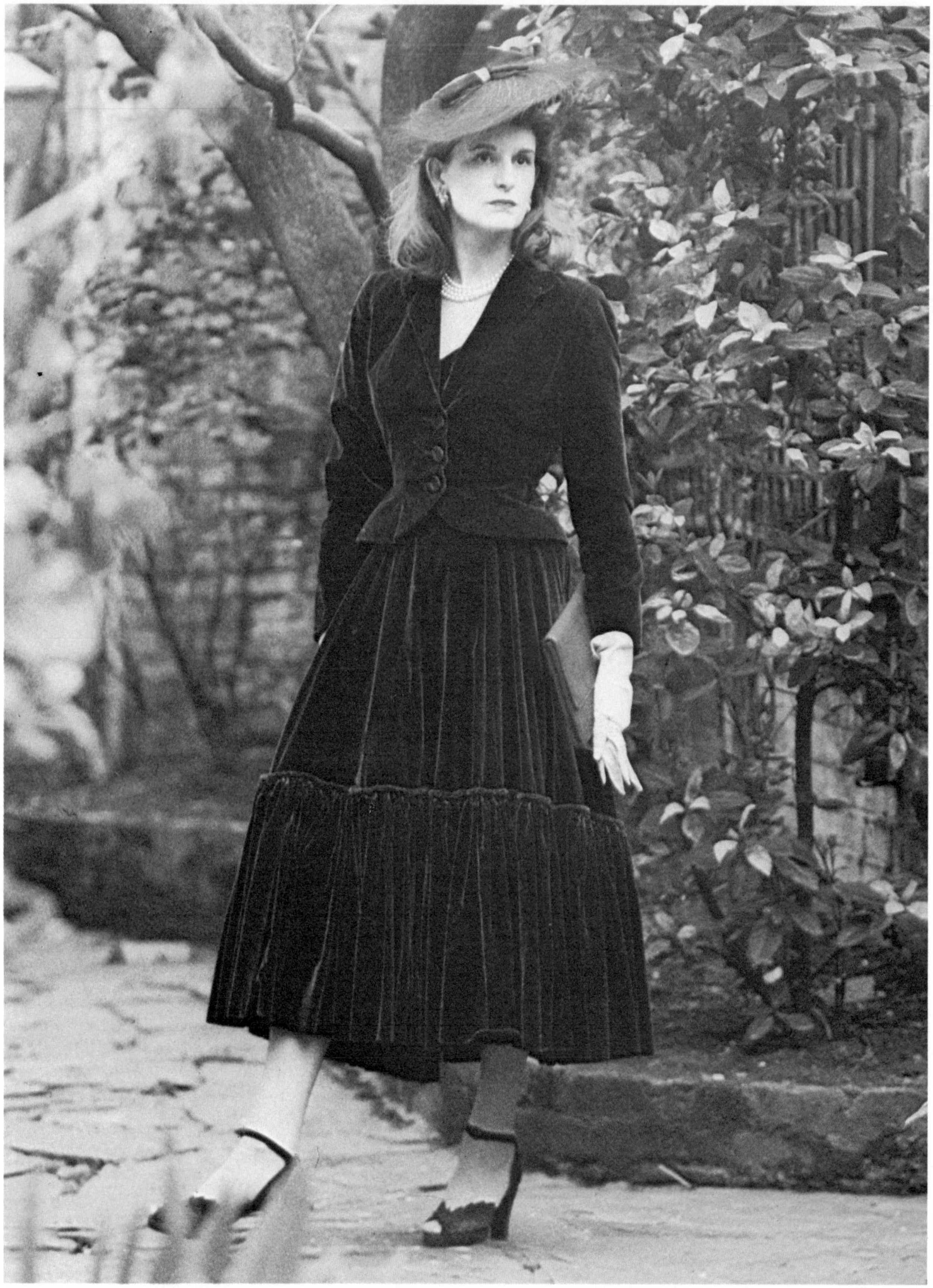

The new look encouraged an abundant use of materials in the following years; on the opposite page is a Lanvin-Castillo satin evening dress made for Vivien Leigh in 1956, embroidered in chenille beads and sequins. Over the page can be seen an American cocktail dress worn in 1960 by Mistinguette, the celebrated French music hall artiste; it is composed of multi-coloured sequins on cream nylon.

1956

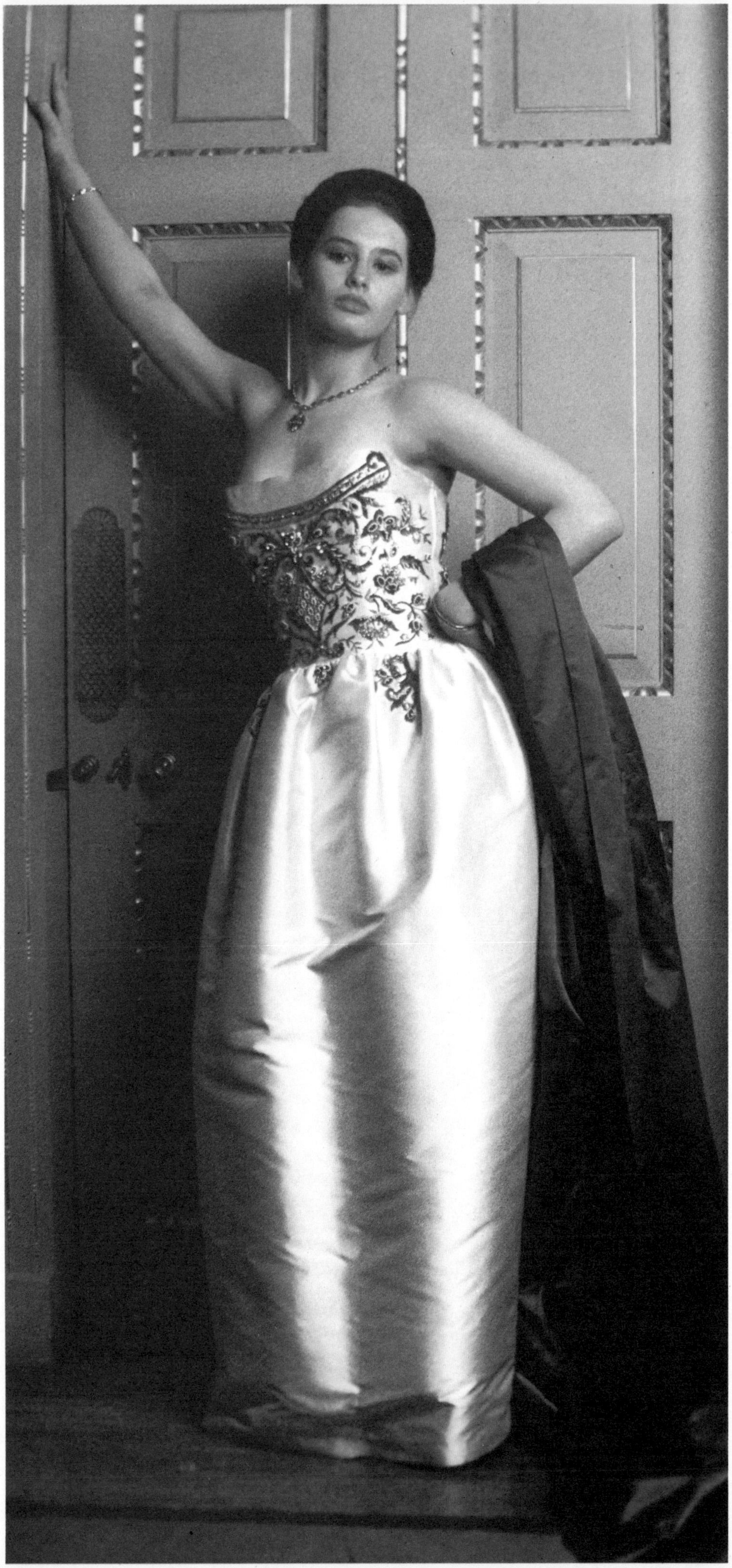

1960

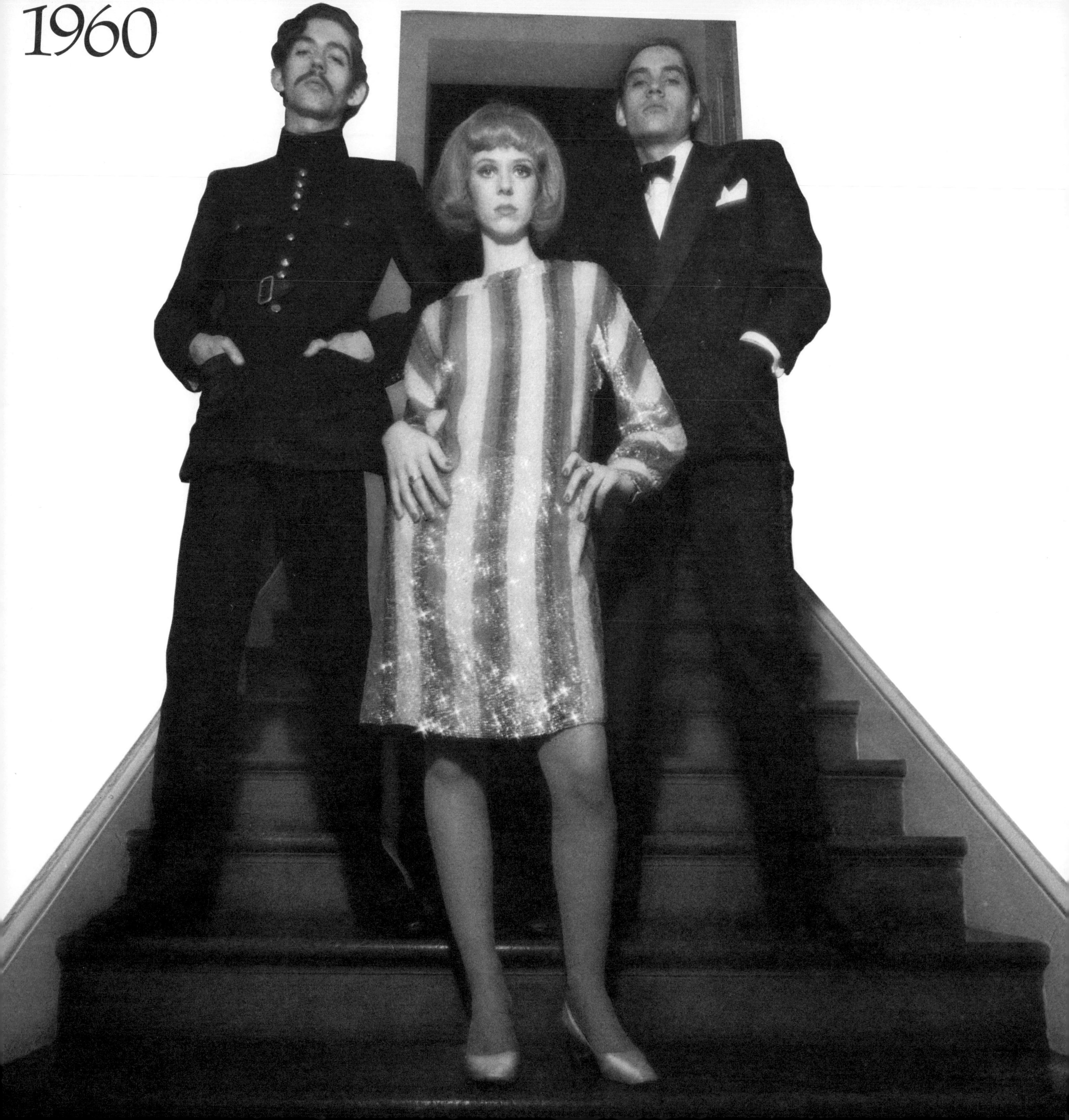

Acknowledgements

Curator: Richard Robson.

Costume gallery staff:
Charles Atkinson, Mary House, Margaret Knopp, Edward Maeder, Doreen Palmer, May Walton, Joan White.

Models: Muriel Appleby, Scenie Arthur, Karan Bowen, Francesca Brindley, Howard Burnham, Jane Charteris, Gill Dark, Deborah Dossor, Georgina Haynes, Nick Howard, Simon Howard, Edmond Lamb, Valerie Lamb, Terri Lawler, Hadyn Maude, Maureen Mercer, Anne Naylor, Jane Olsen, Richard Robson, Fiona Ross, Margaret Ross, Louise Rowe, Mellanie Rowe, Claire Simpson, Penelope Wilson.

Hairdressing and makeup:
Carol Cooper, Margaret Leonard, Pam Meagher, Eileen Mair, Charles Skaife.

Design: Adrian Knowles.

Photography: Naruhito.

Text: Nicholas Howard.

Printing: Ben Johnson and Co Ltd.

The text is set Diatronic Palatino, 11 key minus one on 5¼mm. The paper is Mellotex smooth super white 135 gsm.